OPTIMIZE YOUR BODY, HEAL YOUR MIND

· ·

An Integrative, Innovative, and Powerful

New Protocol for Mental Wellbeing

Dr. Janelle Louis ND

Optimize Your Body, Heal Your Mind: An Integrative, Innovative, and Powerful New Protocol for Mental Wellbeing.

Cover photo by Jeff Louis
Published by Focus Enterprises Publications, an imprint of Focus Enterprises LLC. Printed in the United States of America.

This book contains advice and information relating to healthcare. It is not intended to replace medical advice and should be used to supplement rather than replace regular care by your doctor. It is recommended that you seek your physician's advice before embarking on any medical program or treatment. All efforts have been made to ensure the accuracy of the information contained in this book as of the date of publication. The publisher and the author disclaim liability for any medical outcomes that may occur as a result of applying the methods described in this book. The statements in this book have not been evaluated by the FDA.

Throughout this book, cases of individual patients are referenced. In order to protect patient identities, some identifiers such as patient names, ages, and other identifiers have been changed. Patient symptoms, diagnoses, drug class of active medication, treatment methodology, outcomes, and other relevant details have been preserved.

Publisher's Cataloging-in-Publication Data
Names: Louis, Janelle Aisha, author.
Title: Optimize your body, heal your mind: an integrative, innovative, and powerful new protocol for mental wellbeing / Dr. Janelle Louis ND.
Description: Includes bibliographical references. | Mission, KS: Focus Enterprises Publications, imprint of Focus Enterprises LLC, 2018.
Identifiers: ISBN 9780998350196 | LCCN 2018906646
Subjects: LCSH Mind and body. | Health. | Medicine and psychology. | Mental healing. | Holistic medicine. | Self-care, Health. | Conduct of life. | BISAC HEALTH & FITNESS / Diseases / Nervous System (incl. Brain) | HEALTH & FITNESS / Alternative Therapies
Classification: LCC RA776.5 .L67 2018 | DDC 613--dc23

OPTIMIZE YOUR BODY, HEAL YOUR MIND

An Integrative, Innovative, and Powerful
New Protocol for Mental Wellbeing

Contents

. . . .

To my mother, Karen, whose hard work, dedication, drive, and optimism have taught me to persevere and have faith, and who had faith in what I could do and be, even when I didn't.

To my husband and son, the best supporters
a woman could ever imagine.

Preface

AT THE BEGINNING OF my second year in medical school, I was doing a needs analysis survey as a part of a group in a local community when I met a young man. I'll call him Grant. When I asked Grant about the needs of the community, he told me that the majority of people from age fourteen onward were addicted to cocaine and that if we could do something to help them, that would really meet a grave need. I couldn't help but wonder if these people were self-medicating to address an underlying mental health concern.

I later worked with two doctors who were doing amazing work that focused on addiction medicine and treated individuals with dual diagnoses (a substance abuse disorder and at least one other mental health diagnosis) using pharmaceutical medications in conjunction with integrative therapies.

I did similar work in helping people with dual diagnoses at two additional recovery clinics and, throughout my experiences at these three clinics, I saw both the power of and the great need for an integrative approach to mental and overall wellbeing.

When I started my private practice, I saw this power and need even more clearly as I communicated with and treated my patients. I was constantly researching, engaging in continuing education, and treating my patients using some of the most cutting edge, innovative, and integrative therapies and evaluations available for the treatment of mental health disorders.

As I continued to treat my patients, I began to see a pattern. I saw the same factors at play over and over again, even in patients who carried different mental health diagnoses. I compiled this information and constructed the P7 Protocol™, an integrative, innovative, and powerful new protocol for mental and overall wellbeing. I later decided to write a book about my method. *Optimize Your Body, Heal Your Mind* is the result.

As you'll see when you read the chapter on my personal story, this protocol and book have been a long time in the making.

I wrote this book in order to share my method and to educate the general public about the research surrounding the seldom-suspected factors that significantly impact mental health. I also wrote it to clear up the misconceptions and preconceived notions that I heard time and time again in the expressed thoughts of my patients.

I truly believe that all health concerns have one or more causative factor(s), and that, in many cases, mental health disorders are the result of physiological concerns, such as dysregulation of the immune system as a result of stressful experiences during childhood, hormonal imbalances, genetic and epigenetic predispositions, or other physiological concerns. When we understand the cause of the physiological imbalance, then we are better equipped to address the imbalance and, when we do this, the body is better able to return to a state of optimal wellness.

I believe the P7 Protocol™ has the potential to make a significant impact on the lives of many people, including yours.

As you read this book, I recommend that you read it in chronological order. Many of the topics build upon each other and you may find yourself lost if you skip around.

I also recommend that you come to the research I'll be sharing with an open mind and that you think critically. When it comes to taking control of your health, one of the most important things you can do is ask yourself (and others) why. Never be satisfied with superficial answers or low-quality "studies" (you'll learn how to spot these in chapter eleven; don't worry).

Now that you understand my motivation behind writing *Optimize Your Body, Heal Your Mind* and the potential that it has to change your life, and you're prepared to adopt the mindset necessary to obtain maximum benefit from this book, let's begin our journey.

Introduction

I<small>F YOU'RE READING THIS</small> book, then you likely fall into one of four categories of people:

1. Maybe you've never actually been given a psychiatric diagnosis, but you've realized recently (or maybe you've always known) that something isn't right with your mental health.

2. Maybe you've been diagnosed with a mental health concern and prescribed medication, but you discontinued the medication almost immediately because you didn't like the way it made you feel.

   Perhaps you never even followed through by filling your prescription, because it didn't align with your philosophy of healing. Maybe you tried to see a therapist because of your desire to utilize a more psychotherapeutic approach, but you just couldn't connect with your therapist or it didn't seem to help as much as you had hoped. Now your symptoms are worsening. You need to address your issues, but you don't know where to turn next.

3. Maybe you've been diagnosed with a psychiatric condition and you're taking medication for it. The medication helped initially and you were able to live your life normally again for some time, but lately you've noticed that your symptoms are intensifying despite the fact that there have been no changes to your medication. Maybe they've intensified to the point that you feel your mental health is worse now than it was before you started the medication, and you want to find a way to address your symptoms so that you no longer need to take the medication. Or maybe your medication is still helping tremendously, but you're concerned about the side-effects you're experiencing and the potential long-term effects of the medication.

4. Maybe you have a friend or a loved one who is battling a mental health condition. It hurts you so

much to see them struggling and all you want to be able to do is help them.

Regardless of which category you fall into, you've come to the realization that you cannot accomplish your goals on your own; you need additional help, beyond what your primary care provider or psychiatrist can provide or is providing.

In my private practice, I help patients like you address their mental health concerns by uncovering, identifying, and addressing other aspects of their health that are contributing to their poor mental health. Because many of my patients expressed frustration with the conventional medical community, I began to ask myself how we got here.

In other words, how did we as a society find ourselves in a situation where patients don't feel that they are listened to and where, when a person reports a symptom, we do little or no objective testing in order to identify the cause, instead giving them a psychoactive drug and sending them on their way?

When I began to study the development of the field of psychiatry, it all made sense. I understood the attempts at reform that had been made when the then-standard biological model—a model where a person's poor health was seen as a biological illness and exclusively treated by medical means—was replaced with the revolutionary biopsychosocial model. While not without flaws, this model seeks to help practitioners to think about patients not just as organisms with diseases, but as individual beings whose mental, physical, and social aspects interact with each other resulting in complex behaviors and emotions, all of which affect their overall health. I also understood that when psychiatrists attempt to adopt and truly implement unconventional approaches, they are met with significant roadblocks such as differences in reimbursement rates for prescribing medication versus counseling their patients.[1]

I realized that our current model needs reform, and in my private practice I set out to implement the changes that I wanted to see in the medical community at large. As I continued to treat my patients, I saw that change was possible, that we really could address mental health conditions using a functional approach that utilizes objective testing to gather information about the nature of each concern as well as its contributing factors.

And we could do all of that if we truly spent time with our patients, taking their histories and listening to their stories; taking a comprehensive view of the whole person, including the physical, mental, spiritual, and social aspects of their lives (which are actually all inseparably connected, though we separate them when discussing them in order to facilitate clarity); analyzing how each aspect affects the others; addressing any imbalances in a minimally-invasive manner that helps the body to return to a state of equilibrium; addressing habits and lifestyle factors that may be contributing to a sub-optimal state of wellbeing; and processing emotions and past traumatic experiences in a manner that is both productive and healing.

In my experience, I've seen that it takes hard work, determination, perseverance, and significant investments of time and effort, but it is, in all actuality, possible to optimize your body and heal your mind using an integrative approach.

I'm committed to helping you reach your wellness goals so that you can get back to living life on your own terms. I am convinced that you can regain your freedom—freedom from apprehension, depression, fear, and side-effects—and

I'm committed to helping you overcome the barriers that are holding you back from becoming the person you were meant to be. Through empowering you to take ownership of your own health, I'm committed to helping you live up to the potential that others and I see in you.

CHAPTER ONE

Panic Attacks, An Insensitive Psychiatrist, and the Healing Path

. . . .

My Personal Journey

"WHOEVER IS TELLING YOU to get off of this medication does not love you!" my mother's psychiatrist fumed at her as I stared blankly at him from my seat on the couch across the room. His piercing stare, which was fixed on my mom, was interrupted only by a quick, suspicious glance in my direction.

How did we get here? And why was he so angry? Well, it all started years ago. Many years ago…

Growing up on the island of Trinidad, my early years were pretty interesting. A few years into my mother's marriage, things got really stressful. Without going into all of the details, I'll just say she was dealing with a lot. She was probably about 26 when the stress began, and these stressful circumstances continued until she divorced my father around age 34. My brother was born when things were still fine with her marriage, but my sister and I were born when things were pretty tumultuous.

My Mom's Story

As a result of everything that was going on, my mom battled intense anxiety and depression. My mom's anxiety and depression were characterized by weakness, so much so that she would try to go to the bathroom to bathe, but would be overcome with anxiety and would need to hurry back to her bed for fear that she would collapse on the floor.

I remember seeing my mom lying on her bed, unable to stand for long periods of time. She was so debilitated by her anxiety and depression that she was unable to do much for herself. Oftentimes, I'd come home from school to find my grandmother sponge-bathing my mother or using a bedpan to wash her hair, because my mom was extremely weak and couldn't do these things for herself.

My mom also experienced severe panic attacks in my early years. Her panic attacks generally lasted 5-10 minutes, but they were so intense that, each time, she just knew she was going to die. They would start by what's known as phantosmia or olfactory hallucination; my mom would usually smell a scent that other people didn't smell as a prodromal symptom to her panic attacks. This scent usually took the form of roasting coffee beans or of something burning. She would then experience back and shoulder pain and a sensation as though she had gotten sand in her eyes. Next, her heart would start racing and she would start experiencing nausea, hyperventilation, and difficulty breathing. She would feel cold on the inside and hot on the outside, and she would start shivering. All of this was accompanied by intense fear and the certainty that she would not make it through this attack alive.

Because she never knew when she would experience a panic attack, my mom lived in constant fear of going out into public places alone. This fear of panic attacks led to a worsening of her anxiety and depression, which then led to an increase in the frequency of her panic attacks, and the vicious cycle continued.

One day in Trinidad, my mom was riding on a bus. She was taking my brother to have surgery and her mood was depressed because she had to do this alone. In the midst of feeling extremely stressed out, she began to experience the onset of a panic attack. All of the usual symptoms ensued. She began to experience difficulty breathing, shivering, and a general feeling of weakness.

My mom had learned that eating or drinking something at the onset of a panic attack helped the weak feeling to resolve, but she looked in her bag and she didn't have any food with her. The bus stopped, and my mom shouted, "Does anyone have any water?"

A gentleman on her bus happened to have some frozen rainwater with him, so he gave it to my mom. She drank it as quickly as possible and her panic attack began to subside.

The Appointment That Changed it All

One day, my mom visited our family physician in Trinidad. He sat and spoke with her for a long period of time, explaining to her that her conventional lab results were all within the optimal range and that, if we were going by the numbers, she would have been one of his healthiest patients. Both our physician and my mother, however, knew that she wasn't well.

After a bit more discussion, our physician said something interesting to my mother. He asked, "Do you have any family members in the United States?"

He explained that he believed that hypothalamic-pituitary-adrenal axis dysregulation was the most likely cause of her mental health concerns. In other words, he believed that her poor mental health was a direct result of her high stress levels and prolonged elevation of cortisol, the stress hormone. He believed that my mom was in dire need of a change of environment.

Providentially, my mom had just been invited to the United States to attend my aunt's wedding. Depressed and not feeling up to it, she had declined the invitation, but after speaking with our physician, she called my aunt and let her know that she would be in attendance.

Life in the United States

To make a long story shorter, my mom did attend my aunt's wedding and she ended up staying and attending school here in the United States. My siblings and I eventually came to be with my mom as well. Now, fast-forward a few years. My mom is happily remarried and is mostly free from anxiety, depression, and panic attacks. Life for my mom is great. After a few years, however, changing life circumstances and a new life stressor would lead to a return of her generalized anxiety disorder.

My mom started seeing a psychiatrist who put her on medication to manage her symptoms. Before we realized what was happening, my mom had been on three different psychotropic medications for about two years, and whereas she was only experiencing anxiety when she first started seeing the psychiatrist, she was now experiencing anxiety, depression, and panic attacks which were far more frequent and longer-lasting than they were before she started taking the medication.

My mom shared this with me and expressed her desire to discontinue her medication, so I went with her to see her psychiatrist. And there we were, sitting in his office…

After insinuating that someone was telling my mom that she needed to discontinue her medication and shooting a suspicious glance in my direction, her psychiatrist continued to explain himself.

"You need this medicine to function. I am not treating anxiety and depression; I am preventing them," he stated, visibly exerting great effort to maintain his composure.

He continued to explain to my mom why she needed to continue taking her medication, in spite of the fact that she felt worse on the medication than she felt before she started taking them.

"Well, do you at least have a support group that you could connect me with? I think I would benefit from therapy or a support group," my mom said, to which he responded that he did not know of any therapists or support groups that she could connect with or join.

As I'm mentally revisiting this day, I can't help but chuckle at how unbelievable this interaction sounds. I'm so grateful that since this day, I've had the privilege of meeting so many wonderful, open-minded physicians and psychiatrists who are willing to keep up with the latest research and whose main goals are working together with other relevant practitioners to achieve optimal patient outcomes.

Before leaving the office, my mom reiterated her desire to discontinue her medication, and finally, as we were preparing to leave, her psychiatrist blurted out the information we had been waiting for:

"If you want to get off the medication, it's simple. Cut the tablets in half and take ½ of each tablet, then take ¼ of each tablet, and then you'll be able to discontinue your medication."

My mom and I left the office, happy to have received the coveted weaning protocol and excited to implement it. But it wasn't as easy as we had hoped…

Discontinuation Dilemmas

Concerned about the effects of weaning off of all three medications at the same time, my mom decided to follow the protocol, but wean off of one drug at a time instead of simultaneously weaning off of all three. She began the process and was able to discontinue the first drug, a serotonin-specific reuptake inhibitor (SSRI), by following the psychiatrist's protocol. It was then time for the second.

Excited by the possibility of soon being medication-free, my mom began the weaning process for her second drug, an aminoketone. After beginning the weaning process, she quickly realized that this one would not be as "easy" as the first.

Being the strong and considerate woman that she is, my mom tried to push through these symptoms without telling me or anyone else in our family what she was experiencing; she didn't want us to be concerned about her wellbeing, but in all actuality, my mom was very afraid.

She came to me one night while weaning off of the medication and told me where her life insurance policy information was located. I became bothered and upset that she was sharing this information with me. I had just turned 19 years old and was incredibly uncomfortable with the idea of me needing to contact my mother's life insurance company.

Years later, when my mom reminded me of that incident, she told me that she had been experiencing intense chest and abdominal pain that night and was sure that she would not make it to see the morning. She described the pain as being as intense as the contractions she experienced during childbirth.

In spite of what she was experiencing, I'm grateful that my mom did make it through the night. The following morning, she pulled herself together and went to work. My mom felt extremely weak all day at work and, by the end of the day, she was feeling so terrible that she went to our primary care's office at the end of the day instead of coming straight home like she usually did.

When my mom arrived, she told our primary care physician that she had been experiencing neurological symptoms such as slurred speech, left-sided facial numbness, numbness in her left arm and hand, loss of balance, and difficulty walking. Her systolic blood pressure was also elevated, although she hadn't had any previous history of hypertension. Concerned that she may be having a stroke, our primary care physician told her that they were calling the paramedics to transport her to our local emergency room (ER).

My mom couldn't handle the thought of going to the ER without my step-dad, so she asked them to please let her go home and then have him take her to the ER. Our primary care physician did her very best to persuade my mom to go via ambulance to the ER, to no avail. My mom reasoned within herself that she did feel somewhat better than she felt the night before and if she didn't die then, she probably wouldn't die on her way home.

The doctor had her sign a medical release form and my mom left to go home. When I got home, my dad was preparing to take my mom to the ER. I could tell that my mom was a lot more concerned about the way she was feeling than her words were communicating, and this concerned me greatly. Although it was already late and I needed to be at my university early the following morning, I insisted that I was coming along.

In the Emergency Room

When we arrived at the ER, my mom was seen rather quickly. Her sudden onset of stroke-like symptoms led to her being prioritized over many of the other people in the waiting room.

It wasn't until they came out, put my mom on a stretcher, and quickly wheeled her away to a room that I became keenly aware of my surroundings. All of a sudden, as they were taking my mother away, I noticed the concerned faces of the people in the waiting room. I noticed the characteristic hospital smell. I noticed the look on my dad's face. And I noticed within myself, for the first time, a keen sense of discomfort and dislike associated with being at the hospital.

My dad and I were permitted to accompany my mom to her room and some time after her intake, vitals, and other preliminary procedures, we were informed that the ER medical team believed that the most likely causative factor in my mom's sudden onset of symptoms was her withdrawing too quickly from her medication. They encouraged her to resume taking her full dosage of her medication.

My mom and I were confused, because she had followed her psychiatrist's instructions very carefully, but, after her discharge, we later learned that the weaning protocol was much too fast and that, if there was any hope of weaning off of the medication in as uneventful a manner as possible, we would need to find and implement another, much slower protocol.

Why This Time Was Different

Although I had seen my mom weak and debilitated by her poor mental health when I was a child, there was something different about seeing my mom being wheeled away on a stretcher that day in the ER. I'm still unable to definitively verbalize all of the reasons why, but my experience in the ER that day was very traumatic. It was categorically different from the experiences I had had in early childhood.

I believe it may be because, in spite of my mother being debilitated by her mental state in my youth, she would always push through. I remember power walking with my mom and my siblings up the hill by our home in Trinidad as we repeated after my mom, chanting, "I must, I must, I must improve my health." Even amidst what seemed like an immensely hopeless situation, my mom exhibited hope, faith, and perseverance.

My mom would always, always push through. She would always find ways to overcome the hand that life had dealt her, and I admired her for that. I still do. But that day in the ER, I saw my mom in an entirely different light. I saw her as vulnerable. I saw her as powerless. I saw her as helpless. For the very first time in my teenage life, I saw my mom as human. And that terrified me.

How Trauma Inspired Change

You know the old adage: out of ashes, beauty comes. In the midst of the traumatic experience of my mom being in the hospital, I began to think about the direction of my life.

I had wanted to be a physician since I was six years old. I had never really desired to be anything else. I focused all of my education and extra-curricular activities toward that goal. When my mom was in the hospital, however, I became somewhat disillusioned with the medical profession. I began to feel like my mom's medication and her psychiatrist had failed her.

I started to think that, like our family physician in Trinidad had implied, surely there must be a physiological reason why she was experiencing these psychiatric symptoms; and surely there must be a way to address her mental health without using medication that would lead to an intensification of her symptoms, while creating chemical dependencies in the brain such that trying to separate herself from them results in stroke-like symptoms warranting emergency hospitalization. I wondered why the doctors had not been able to uncover the cause of my mom's symptoms, and for some time I put the idea of becoming a physician on hold. I began to reconsider my career path.

After the Hospital Scene

After my mom was discharged, she and I were able to find a slower, more appropriate weaning protocol online and she was eventually able to successfully discontinue her aminoketone. Two down, one to go. My mom had strategically chosen the order in which she would discontinue her medication. She had accurately hypothesized that discontinuing her benzodiazepine would be the most difficult, so she had saved that one for last.

Throughout the process of weaning off of her benzodiazepine, my mom experienced mental confusion, dizziness, difficulty breathing, and intense weakness each morning that resolved completely at night, only to return the following morning. After more than five months of gradually reducing her dosage, my mom was finally able to discontinue her third and final drug.

Finally Free!

My mom was now medication-free. She reported that the heavy feeling and the dizziness that she had experienced while on and while withdrawing from her medication had resolved. She was still experiencing some anxiety, but, for the most part, she was starting to feel normal again.

This isn't the case for everyone, but after discontinuing her medication, my mom began to experience a dramatic reduction in symptoms. She reported mental clarity and a resolution of her dizziness. For the most part, she stopped having panic attacks and, instead of existing in a constant state of anxiety, my mom's mood dramatically improved. She still experienced some anxious feelings when facing life stressors, but it was nothing like what she had experienced before.

My Next Step

By the time my mom finished weaning off of her medication, I had graduated from my university. I was unclear on the next step to take as far as a career was concerned, but I knew that, if I did pursue my dream to become a doctor, I wanted to approach things differently. I truly believed that every health condition had at least one definite cause, and I wanted to be the type of doctor who would search for and address the underlying cause of disease, working with the body by giving it everything that it needs in order to facilitate healing.

It was around that time that I discovered naturopathic medicine. I knew immediately that this was the type of medicine that I wanted to practice. Providentially, I also met a naturopathic doctor who had graduated from the school I was interested in at that time, and she helped to address some of my questions and concerns as well. To make a long story shorter, I applied to naturopathic medical school, was accepted, and moved across the country to pursue my dream.

While in medical school, much of my training was geared toward treating mental illness. This was unintentional at first. In spite of my extensive personal, family experience on the receiving end of psychiatry, I was actually drawn to obstetrics and midwifery. My earliest clinical experiences, however, which involved treating individuals battling substance abuse disorders, anxiety, depression, panic attacks, bipolar disorder, disordered eating, and other mental health concerns, further opened my eyes to the widespread need in the field of psychiatry for more practitioners who provide empathetic, compassionate, and individualized care that sees the whole person and not just a diagnosis, and that seeks to uncover and address the underlying cause of each individual's health concerns.

I made up my mind pretty early on that I wanted to help address mental health concerns, and I tailored as much as possible of my education, clinical training, and life experiences toward this goal.

How My Education Helped My Mom

While I was in medical school, my mom was caring for my beloved, elderly grandmother. Over seventeen years had elapsed since the time when my grandmother used to care for my mom while she was overwhelmed with anxiety and depression and now the roles were reversed. My grandmother had grown much older since then and she now met the criteria for and was diagnosed with "probable Alzheimer's disease," another condition I am passionate about addressing in my private practice.

My mom was one of my grandmother's two main caregivers, and although caring for my grandmother was therapeutic for her, she did worry about what the future held for my grandmother. Around this time, my grandmother also had to have emergency surgery as a result of complications from another health concern. These factors, in addition to working a stressful new job and dealing with other resurfacing life stressors took a toll on my mom and she began to experience a return of her anxiety.

This time, however, I was able to use the knowledge and clinical experience that I had gained in medical school to help my mother modulate her mood and restore balance to her hypothalamic-pituitary-adrenal axis without the use of pharmaceutical medication. By following my recommendations, my mom was able to manage her stressors in a manner that was productive and not destructive, and she was eventually able to do so on her own, without daily medication or supplementation. Today in my private practice, this is my goal for all of my patients.

CHAPTER TWO

From Exorcisms to Eclectic Wisdom

. . . .

The History of Psychiatric Treatment in America

*"The more I learn, the more I realize
how much I don't know."*

THIS STATEMENT, OFTEN CREDITED to Albert Einstein, echoes my sentiments when I think about the human brain. Our brains are incredibly complicated structures. The brain can be thought of as a complex system, a network of some sort, which enacts changes within the body (and life) as a result of interactions between the various players involved in the system. These players include genetics, neurotransmitters like dopamine and serotonin, hormones, neural behavior, neuroplasticity, and many others.

The brain's complexity has a definite impact on the field of psychiatry. Because we haven't been able to positively identify and do not currently understand all of the factors at play in the development of any of the mental health disorders, it has been difficult to develop appropriate diagnostics. In this regard, the field of psychiatry is notably different from every other field of medicine and presents its own unique challenges.

To date, unlike physical diseases like diabetes and hypertension, there is no blood test or physical exam that can definitively confirm that a person has schizophrenia, bipolar disorder, or any other mental health concern. As a result, we currently make psychiatric diagnoses by going through a series of diagnostic criteria and assessing whether or not the patient meets the criteria for a given disorder. Psychiatrists and other relevant professionals have constructed these criteria to the best of their ability using what we know about the clinical presentation of each mental health disorder; however, the fact that there aren't many objective diagnostic tests does dramatically increase the rate of misdiagnosis.

For example, a survey conducted in the year 2000 revealed that a striking 69% of individuals who were eventually diagnosed with bipolar disorder were initially misdiagnosed. Those who were misdiagnosed actually saw an average of four different physicians before obtaining their current diagnosis. The individuals surveyed were mostly happy with their current treatment plans, but for more than one-third of them, it took over 10 years before they were finally diagnosed and able to receive proper treatment.[2]

The Diagnostic and Statistical Manual of Mental Disorders, which is the book that contains the diagnostic criteria for all psychiatric and mental health concerns, explicitly states that in order to meet the criteria for most mental health disorders, the symptoms must not be due to the use of a mind-altering substance (with the exception of substance abuse disorders, of course) and must not be better explained by another physiological illness. When adhered to, this limits the rate of misdiagnosis somewhat and encourages doctors to search for and identify any underlying physiological factors that may be causing or contributing to patients' poor mental health.

Psychiatry In The Early Years

The field of psychiatry didn't always have these safeguards in place to reduce the rate of misdiagnosis and mistreatment among those dealing with poor mental health. We have undoubtedly come a long way. I'll explain.

The term "psychiatry" didn't come about until the 1800s. Prior to the 19th century, most people viewed mental illness as a spiritual affliction or "demon possession."

Imagine this scene with me: it's a Sunday afternoon in the early 1700s and we are in the mood for entertainment. All of a sudden we see a flyer for a local attraction. From this flyer, we learn that for a small fee, we can head down to the local hospital and be entertained by the "mad men" and "mad women" (those suffering from mental illness) who were chained and raving in the hospital basement.[3]

Before the 19th century, the mentally ill were seen as fierce and dangerous and the treatment at that time involved forcing them into submission by tying them down, chaining them to things, or otherwise restraining them, and beating and whipping them into submission. They were treated like creatures lower than animals whose wills needed to be broken.

The Advent of Modern Psychiatry

During the late 1700s, two distinct schools of thought began to develop regarding the cause of mental illness. While the vast majority of people still saw mental illness as a spiritual problem, a Scotland-educated doctor by the name of Benjamin Rush began to work to change this belief. Known as the father of American psychiatry, Dr. Rush was the first person to believe and advocate that mental illness was a disease of the mind.[4]

Dr. Rush believed that mental illness came about as a result of circulatory abnormalities in the vessels of the brain, and he believed these circulatory abnormalities could be the result of a wide variety of physical or psychological causes. Unlike other people in his day, Dr. Rush taught that the mentally ill should be treated with respect. He was not, however, completely free from the biases of his European instructors and Dr. Rush was cited on several occasions comparing the mentally ill to animals. Being an academic, he also employed a variety of dangerous and sometimes inhumane "medical treatments" that he had learned in Europe in the treatment of the mentally ill. These treatments included bloodletting, the use of cathartic laxatives and violent emetics, a medical device that Dr. Rush invented and called "the tranquilizing chair," sedatives, and physical restraints.[4,5]

Opposition to the Medical Treatments

These types of "medical treatments" were a common occurrence centuries ago, but there was at least one group of people who did not support this treatment of the mentally ill. In fact, they decided to do something about it.

In the year 1813, dissatisfied with the way those battling mental illness were treated at the local hospital, the Quakers of Pennsylvania founded an institution called the Friends' Asylum for the Relief of Persons Deprived of the Use of Their Reason. The Friends' Asylum was the first private psychiatric hospital in the United States. There, the Quakers used what became known as "moral treatment" to help their patients get well. Moral treatment was founded upon the beliefs that all patients deserved to be treated with dignity and respect, that all patients should be involved in decisions about their care, and that those battling mental health concerns could be cured if they were treated with respect and kindness and if they were put in an environment that was conducive to healing.[3]

Instead of being housed in the damp basement of the local hospital, each patient at the Friends' Asylum was given a room with a window so that they could be exposed to sunlight and fresh air, and they were permitted to work in the garden, which afforded them opportunities for exercise and exposure to green space and nature. They were provided educational programs, and, for entertainment, they were provided opportunities to read, enjoy fine arts by visiting the museum, and engage in other similar activities.

Through the use of moral treatment, many patients were able to regain their mental health and people began to fund other institutions, both private and public, that followed this model. As a general rule, these newer institutions were all kept comparatively small, with 250 patients or fewer, and they produced good results as well. McLean Hospital in Boston and Bloomingdale Asylum in New York reported that approximately 60% of all admitted patients were discharged as cured/recovered, much improved, or improved. The Friends' Asylum had a track record of 50%

of all admitted patients being discharged as cured as a result of the moral treatment offered there.[5]

The Struggle for Power

As the "hospitals" that used moral treatment became increasingly successful at helping people to regain their mental health, physicians began to take note. Most of the asylums founded in the 1810s were run by non-medical superintendents or by physicians who did not approve of the dangerous "medical treatments" that were commonly used. The medical profession had no choice but to acknowledge that the average physician played a minor role, if any at all, in the asylum model of psychiatry.[5]

To combat this perceived threat, members of the Connecticut State Medical Society devised a plan. They built a local asylum and included within its bylaws a clause that stated that its superintendent had to be a physician, and, in 1824, the Hartford Retreat was founded.[5]

Although somewhat similar, this institution was different from the other asylums. It would utilize both moral treatment and the medical treatments of the day in order to provide what they referred to as superior care to the mentally ill.

Groups of physicians in other states began to follow the Connecticut State Medical Society's lead and other asylums were erected. Physicians were elected to serve as medical superintendents and both moral treatment and medical treatments were practiced at these institutions. Gradually, the medical treatments began to increase in proportion to the moral treatment and this was the beginning of moral treatment's downfall.

An Unforeseen Calamity

Another factor that led to the downfall of moral treatment was something that was a bit less predictable. A woman by the name of Dorothea Dix who had benefitted from the moral treatment in her own personal life made it her business to see to it that this type of care would be made available to people struggling with mental health concerns across the country. She traveled to different states and engaged legislators, exposing the atrocities of how the mentally ill were being treated in their jurisdictions. As a direct result of her efforts, twenty states either built or enlarged psychiatric hospitals[5].

To fill these large, new hospitals, people with a variety of different types of illnesses that weren't previously treated at the asylums, such as neurosyphilis, brain tumors, and senile dementia, were admitted. With the loss of the small, home-like atmosphere in these state hospitals and with this influx of very diverse patients, it was no longer possible for patients to receive the same level of care and attention. Although they weren't in its truest sense, hospitals still claimed to be practicing moral treatment. As a result, people began to see moral treatment as an archaic ideology that did not work, and its downfall became imminent.[5]

Modern Approaches to Psychiatry◻The proliferation of state-run and private psychiatric hospitals led to the gradual development of psychiatry as we know it—a medical specialty with very little trace of its history of the moral treatment.

In spite of the changes that have taken place throughout the years, it's evident that every major phase of American psychiatry's evolution has had both benefits and drawbacks.

The Dr. Rush era was filled with dangerous medical treatments; however, he believed and advocated that there may be a physiological cause for mental illness. This led to individuals who would come after him searching for and actually identifying a variety of causative and contributing factors to mental illness.

Moral treatment, as practiced by the Quakers, did not rely on much objective laboratory testing or other diagnostic procedures, but from them we learned the importance of the doctor-patient relationship, lifestyle medicine, treating patients with respect and dignity, allowing them to play an active role in their care, and encouraging social responsibility and a renewed perception of oneself.

The era that came afterward eventually phased out many aspects of the moral treatment, including the most beneficial aspects but, at least for some time, it emphasized the importance of merging lifestyle medicine and social responsibility with advanced diagnostics. During this era, physicians, researchers, and scientists were able to identify and develop testing for a variety of causative and contributory factors pertaining to mental illness.

It's impossible to say that any era was absolutely, in all points, superior to another. I believe that the approach that really brings about the best results—and we are seeing more and more of this approach today—is an eclectic approach that takes the best of each era and combines them into a fresh, new (but not really new) model of care. This is the approach that I take, and this is the direction that I believe the future of psychiatry is heading.

CHAPTER THREE

The P7 Protocol™

· · · · · · · · · · · · · · · · · ·

The Missing Link in Modern Psychiatry

IN TAKING AN INTEGRATIVE approach to mental wellness, I've found that there are seven key dimensions that need to be addressed in order to lay the foundation for health and provide the body with what it needs to regain mental and overall wellbeing. My approach to addressing mental health concerns involves addressing these seven dimensions—the seven Ps—through the P7 Protocol™. I've found that, in most cases of suboptimal mental health, addressing these seven dimensions and correcting any deficiencies or dysfunction that exists results in a significant reduction in or complete resolution of symptoms.

The seven Ps of the P7 Protocol™ are Predispositions, Pathways, Profiles, Personalization, Panoptic inventory,

Professionals, and Prescriptions.

Of note is the fact that, although it is at times, completion of the 7 Ps of the P7 Protocol™ is not always linear; each case is different. In fact, I frequently begin by addressing the first P, *Predispositions*, then moving on to *Pathways*, *Profiles*, and *Personalization*, then revisiting *Profiles*, then skipping to *Professionals*, then completing the *Panoptic inventory*, and so on.

We'll discuss each of these Ps in great detail and the role they each play in the successful treatment of mental health conditions over the next seven chapters.

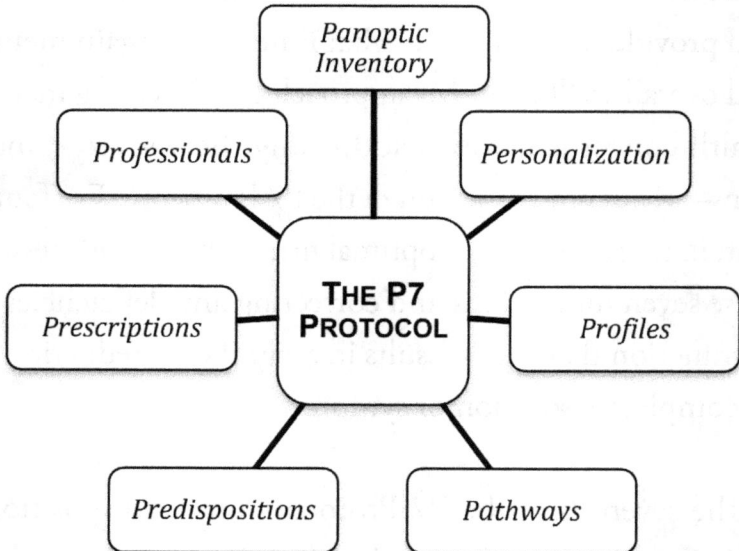

CHAPTER FOUR

Predispositions

· · · · · · · · · · · · · · · · · · ·

How Your Genes Can Make You Blue

I USUALLY BEGIN ADDRESSING A mental health concern at the *Predispositions* section of the P7 Protocol™. I do so by looking at the genetic predispositions to suboptimal mental health that my patient may have. First of all, I want to know how my patient's genetics are impacting his or her ability to produce and to degrade neurotransmitters like dopamine and serotonin.

Here's just one common example: There is a specific gene called the methylene tetrahydrofolate reductase (MTHFR) gene, which contains the DNA required to create the MTHFR enzyme. Before we discuss the importance of this particular gene, let's discuss some background information.

One of the MTHFR enzyme's jobs is to convert synthetic folic acid (which is found in fortified and processed foods like breads, cereals, pasta, and nut milks) to the active form of the vitamin, methylfolate. Methylfolate then helps transform an amino acid called homocysteine into another amino acid called methionine via a process called re-methylation.

Methionine is later converted into a substance called S-adenosylmethionine (SAMe). SAMe is necessary for the production of neurotransmitters like serotonin, dopamine, and epinephrine[6]; therefore, if you aren't getting enough of the active form of vitamin B9, methylfolate, or if, for one reason or another, you aren't able to efficiently convert synthetic folic acid into the active form, this may result in elevated homocysteine levels and suboptimal mental health. This is because preliminary research suggests that elevations in homocysteine are associated with lower levels of dopamine and serotonin and with increased risk for and increased severity of symptoms in depression, post-traumatic stress disorder, bipolar disorder, cognitive deficits, and schizophrenia.[7]

Now let's return to our discussion of the MTHFR gene. A single nucleotide polymorphism (SNP) is a type of genetic variation that reflects a change in one building block of DNA at a specific position in the DNA sequence. There are two common SNPs located in the MTHFR gene—C677T and A1298C. Having these SNPs can lead to your MTHFR enzyme being less active, which can lead to higher levels of homocysteine.[7]

If you have one or more SNPs in this gene, you may have a difficult time converting folic acid to methylfolate. If you have low levels of methylfolate, you may not convert homocysteine into methionine as effectively as people who have the normal variants[7]. If you aren't converting homocysteine to methionine, blood homocysteine levels will begin to rise, there will be lower amounts of methionine, and SAMe will be affected down the line, which will likely affect neurotransmitter production and overall mental health. Clinically, we see a significant correlation between SNPs in the MTHFR gene and the incidence of mental health concerns like depression, bipolar disorder, and schizophrenia.[8]

In looking at my patients' predispositions, not only do I want to know about their MTHFR genetic statuses and other genes that affect neurotransmitter production, degradation, and function, I also want to know how their detoxification pathways are functioning and how their livers metabolize different drugs.

When we come into contact with substances such as pesticides, pharmaceutical medication, alcohol, and food additives, one of the liver's jobs is to convert these substances into non-toxic, water-soluble substances so that they can be excreted from the body through bile, urine, or feces. In order to do this, the liver takes these substances through a two-step detoxification process using a network of enzymes known as the cytochrome P450 (CYP450) system.

The CYP450 system is most notably present in the liver, but also found in small amounts in the small intestines, lungs, placenta, and kidneys where it plays a crucial role in detoxification, among other things.

It isn't uncommon for people to have SNPs in the genes that control the production of the CYP450 enzymes. When SNPs are present, the activity of these enzymes can either be increased, leading to them eliminating these substances from the body much faster than expected, or the activity of these enzymes can be decreased, resulting in them being sluggish and removing the substances from the body much more slowly than expected.

This is particularly important for pharmaceutical medication because if you are prescribed a drug that is metabolized by a specific enzyme in the CYP450 system and you happen to have increased activity at that enzyme (we call this being a rapid metabolizer), then your body will eliminate the drug much more quickly than the average person and you will need a higher dosage in order for the drug to have the same effect compared to if you did not have the SNP in that enzyme. On the other hand, if you are a slow metabolizer and you have decreased activity in a given enzyme, the drug will be eliminated much more slowly and will remain within your body for a much longer period of time, compared to if you did not have a SNP at that enzyme. If you are a slow metabolizer and you are taking a drug that is metabolized through that enzyme, you will need a lower dose than a person who is a normal or rapid metabolizer. If you are a slow metabolizer and the liver is not able to clear the drug as quickly as needed, the result can be a build-up of toxic levels of the drug within your body, or you may experience drug-related side effects at a much lower dose than is expected.[9]

Although the CYP450 system is comprised of over 50 different enzymes, six of them are responsible for metabolizing 90% of drugs prescribed to humans. These enzymes are CYP1A2, CYP2C9, CYP2C19, CYP2D6, CYP3A4, and CYP3A5. Testing for genetic variation in the metabolism of these enzymes can be beneficial in people who are currently on medication, people who are considering taking pharmaceutical medication, and those who were on medication in the past but discontinued due to adverse effects. This is because we are able to predict how well or how poorly you will respond to a given medication based on the variants of CYP450 genes that you have inherited and can select a medication for you that is most likely to address your health concerns and help you start feeling better.

Predispositions & Mental Health – Case Study

Lucille came in to my office with, among other things, concerns of anxiety, some depression, and insomnia, which she said she had been experiencing for the past 6 years or more. She had tried a variety of different medications and was taking Wellbutrin, Xanax, and the maximum dosage of Ambien to help manage her symptoms at the time when she came in to see me. Her symptoms were not well controlled, as her mood and fatigue were significantly impacting her ability to complete her activities of daily living.

In analyzing Lucille's predispositions, I discovered that she was a heterozygous carrier and had inherited one copy of the C677T MTHFR SNP, resulting in her enzyme exhibiting about 35% reduced activity.[10] I also discovered that she was an ultra-rapid metabolizer of one of the main CYP450 enzymes that metabolized Ambien. This explained why she was still experiencing insomnia on the maximum dosage; her body was eliminating the drug much more quickly than expected, so she would have needed a higher dose than a person who exhibited normal enzymatic metabolism in order to achieve the same results. Having looked at the way in which her body metabolized drugs, we now had the information we needed to make recommendations for a different sleep aid, should it be necessary.

In order to support Lucille's MTHFR enzymatic activity and to compensate for the deficiencies caused by her reduced enzyme activity, I had Lucille supplement with the active form of folate, as well as other B vitamins and cofactors. Because her insomnia was related to her anxiety,

I hypothesized that addressing her anxiety would indirectly help address her insomnia. I also addressed Lucille's other concerns.

When Lucille returned to my office four weeks later, she was happy to report significant improvements in her mood and overall quality of life. She reported that her anxiety had significantly decreased and that her sleep had improved dramatically. She had been able to decrease both her Xanax and her Ambien dosages by half. Any depression she was experiencing was minimal.

This is just one example of how looking at genetic predispositions can help inform treatment of mental health disorders. There are many other genes that influence mental health. Evaluating for these genetic variations and compensating for them when necessary really does go a long way toward improving quality of life, even in cases where people have tried a variety of different pharmaceutical medications and experienced little relief.

CHAPTER FIVE

Pathways

· · · · · · · · · · · · · · · · · ·

Don't Forget the Glands in Your Plans

IN ADDRESSING THE SECOND P in the P7 Protocol™, *Pathways*, I look at a variety of different factors. At this point, I am most interested in the biochemical pathways within the body that can significantly impact mental health. These include the pathways for steroid hormone production, where I look at hormones like estrogen, testosterone, progesterone, and their metabolites; thyroid hormones and other markers of thyroid function; peptide hormones like insulin and other markers of glycemic control; the hypo-thalamic-pituitary-adrenal axis which involves hormones like cortisol, epinephrine, and norepinephrine, among others; indicators of neurotransmitter function; and more.

Many of these biochemical pathways begin with the hypothalamus, which is a region of the forebrain that coordinates the activities of a very important gland in the brain, the pituitary gland. The hypothalamus connects our nervous systems with our endocrine systems by sending hormone messengers to the pituitary gland in order to cause it to start producing and secreting hormones. The pituitary gland then sends hormone messengers to various glands throughout the body in order to cause them to produce and secrete their hormones. We refer to these pathways as the hypothalamic-pituitary-X axis, with X being the endocrine gland that produces hormones at the third level in the pathway.

For example, so far I've mentioned the hypothalamic-pituitary-adrenal (HPA) axis in reference to the stress response. In this pathway, the hypothalamus secretes corticotropin-releasing hormone, which causes the pituitary gland to release adrenocorticotropic hormone (ACTH), a hormone whose primary function is to stimulate the secretion of the stress hormone cortisol. ACTH may also increase the production of enzymes that result in an increase in other adrenal hormones, such as epinephrine and norepinephrine.[11]

This is how the HPA axis works, and the other axes follow a similar model of a releasing hormone being secreted by the hypothalamus, leading to a stimulating hormone being secreted by the pituitary gland, which then leads to the gland that is the target of the stimulating hormone secreting its own hormones into the bloodstream. We'll talk specifically about the hypothalamic-pituitary-gonadal (HPG) axis and the hypothalamic-pituitary-thyroid (HPT) axis, and I'll share the details behind why I look at these two areas.

The HPG Axis – Reproductive Hormone Pathways

In the year 2001, a doctor by the name of Gerald Lincoln noticed that a drop in testosterone levels after mating season led to a behavioral state of nervousness, irritability, lethargy and depression in male animals. To describe this phenomenon, he coined the term "irritable male syndrome."[12] This led to a plethora of research being done on human males to identify whether or not this phenomenon would also be seen in men who had low testosterone levels.

To date, a relationship between declining testosterone levels and major depressive disorder has not been positively identified, but research suggests that the gradual decline in testosterone level seen in aging men may lead to a milder, more chronic form of depression such as dysthymia,[13] which is now referred to clinically as persistent depressive disorder.

The relationship between reproductive hormones and schizophrenia is slightly clearer than that of reproductive hormones and depression. We know that both males and females are most likely to be diagnosed with schizophrenia during late adolescence, and that, throughout their lifetimes, males are at an approximately 40% greater risk of being diagnosed with schizophrenia than women.[14] Researchers believe this may be because estrogen modulates the release of neurotransmitters like dopamine and serotonin in the brain in a manner similar to atypical antipsychotics and therefore offers a protective effect against schizophrenia, whereas, while testosterone may benefit negative symptoms in males with schizophrenia, it may also lead to an increase in male vulnerability to schizophrenia compared to estrogen because it lacks the neuroprotection and neurotransmitter modulation that estrogen offers.[15]

While estrogen generally offers protection against schizophrenia in both genders, fluctuations in reproductive hormones, particularly estrogen, can be a significant contributing factor to mental health disorders in women. Research shows that the time periods when women's estrogen levels are rapidly declining tend to be associated with increased risk of mental health concerns. Clinically, we frequently see anxiety and depression associated with time periods when estrogen is decreasing, such as the luteal phase of the menstrual cycle, the post-partum period, and menopause. We recognize anxiety and depression at these times as pre-menstrual syndrome, pre-menstrual dysphoric disorder, post-partum depression, post-partum anxiety, post-menopausal depression, and post-menopausal anxiety.

We also see reproductive hormones, including fluctuations in estrogen[16] and increases in testosterone,[17] being strongly associated with symptoms of other mental health concerns in women, such as bipolar disorder and psychosis. In fact, one large-scale study involving over 1100 women and over 600 men estimated that women diagnosed with bipolar disorder are more than 23 times more likely to be admitted for reasons related to their bipolar disorder (e.g. depression, mania) during the first month after childbirth when estrogen levels are rapidly declining compared to during their pregnancies when levels are increasing.[18]

The HPG Axis – Case Study

These are just a few of the ways that reproductive hormones can impact mental health. In light of these facts, I take a detailed look into my patients' hormone levels in order to identify any hormonal imbalances that may be contributing to their mental health concerns. Instead of looking at estrogen, testosterone, and progesterone alone, I take a comprehensive look at my patients' hormones including looking at the hormones that are secreted higher up in the HPG axis and the metabolites of these reproductive hormones. Doing so enables me to understand how the hormones are interacting with each other and where in the pathway, if anywhere, a problem is located. The research shows and I've seen in my practice that, in many cases, addressing problems related to the HPG axis actually leads to a decrease or a resolution of psychiatric symptoms. Here's an example:

Joyce was a 50-year-old female who had been treated for depression with a variety of different medications after the birth of her daughter 21 years prior. Most recently, she had been on an aminoketone and an SSRI, but by the time she came in to see me, she had weaned herself off of them both. At that time, she was experiencing pretty severe depression. She reported a lack of interest in things she had previously enjoyed; feeling down, depressed, and hopeless; experiencing difficulty falling asleep, fatigue, and diminished appetite; feeling like she was a failure; and experiencing difficulty concentrating nearly every day over the two weeks that preceded our first appointment together. She had also reported thoughts that she would be better off dead several days over the same time period.

Joyce's symptoms began after the birth of her daughter, at a time when estrogen levels were rapidly declining. Her significant medical history also included having one of her ovaries, the primary source of estrogen production, surgically removed some time after her daughter's birth. Because of these two details, I suspected that Joyce's hormones may have been a significant causative and/or contributing factor to her depression, so I tested her hormones.

What I found was not surprising. Joyce's reproductive hormones were at or below the post-menopausal reference range. Because my philosophy of healing involves using the least invasive methods first and working with the body to give it what it needs in order to address any deficiencies, I made non-invasive, botanical recommendations to help support Joyce's adrenal glands since the adrenal glands produce estrogen and progesterone when the ovaries are no longer able to do so. I also made botanical recommendations to modulate Joyce's reproductive hormone levels and to address her depression and difficulty concentrating.

Due to some logistical issues, it took a few weeks to get Joyce on a personalized treatment plan that worked for her, but two weeks after she implemented the plan I just described, as well as the lifestyle recommendations that I made, she informed me that she had "gotten better." Her depression had significantly decreased and her concentration had dramatically improved. I continued to work with Joyce, adjusting her treatment plan to meet her body's changing needs, and when I last spoke with her, she excitedly reported that she felt that her anxiety levels were decreasing and she was continuing to improve each day.

The HPT Axis – Thyroid Hormone Pathways

Now that I've explained why I check reproductive hormones when seeking to identify underlying contributing factors to mental health concerns, here's why I check the thyroid hormones and run other tests that are relevant to the HPT axis:

The thyroid gland, which is located in the neck just below the Adam's apple, controls the body's growth, metabolism, and development. Having an underactive thyroid gland is referred to as hypothyroidism, while having an overactive thyroid gland is referred to as hyperthyroidism. Symptoms of hypothyroidism include fatigue, cold sensitivity, constipation, dry skin, brittle nails, thinning hair, unexplained weight gain, puffy face, muscle weakness, impaired memory, and depression, while symptoms of hyperthyroidism include fatigue, increased sensitivity to heat, diarrhea or loose stools, brittle hair, insomnia, unexpected weight loss, increased appetite, rapid heart rate, nervousness, anxiety, and irritability.

In the HPT axis, the hypothalamus secretes thyrotropin-releasing hormone (TRH), which causes the pituitary gland to secrete thyroid-stimulating hormone (TSH). When TSH is released into the bloodstream, it travels to the thyroid gland where it tells the thyroid gland to produce and secrete thyroid hormones—thyroxine (T4) and a small amount of triiodothyronine (T3)—into the bloodstream. Some of the T4 is then converted to T3 in other parts of the body.

When screening for thyroid disorders, most doctors only test for TSH. The reference range for TSH varies from lab to lab, but it is generally around 0.45 uIU/ml to around 4.50 uIU/ml. To oversimplify things, if your TSH comes back above the reference range, you have an underactive thyroid or hypothyroidism; and if it comes back below the reference range, then your thyroid is overly active, which would signify hyperthyroidism.

That sounds simple enough: If you have a high TSH then you may be at increased risk for depression because of the hypothyroidism, and if you have a low TSH you may be at increased risk for anxiety because of the hyperthyroidism. There's only one problem: There may be an issue with the reference range for TSH.

The data from some pretty important studies suggest that the reference range for TSH isn't as reliable as we once thought. The authors of a study based on the National Health and Nutrition Examination Survey III looked at the relationships between TSH and two types of thyroid antibodies in pregnant women. At the end of this study, researchers concluded that when we initially looked at thyroid function and came up with the "normal" values for the TSH reference range, we may have been wrong about the upper limit because of certain confounding factors.[19] This means that there may be people with TSH values that are technically considered to be "normal," but who are actually suffering from the symptoms that we see in people who are diagnosed with hypothyroidism.

To build on our understanding of thyroid function, let's consider the autoimmune thyroid disorder, Hashimoto's thyroiditis. Hashimoto's thyroiditis is an autoimmune thyroid disorder where the thyroid gland is being attacked and destroyed by the body's immune system.

In the early stages of Hashimoto's, many people experience symptoms of both hypothyroidism and hyperthyroidism. This is because the immune system's attack on the thyroid gland leads to the T3 and T4 being released from the damaged gland into the bloodstream. This creates a hyperthyroid state. The high T3 and T4 in the blood tell the brain to decrease the TRH and TSH in order to decrease the thyroid hormone secretion. This then leads to a hypothyroid state. This process can repeat itself for some time, resulting in the person reflecting either a hyperthyroid or a hypothyroid state, until the thyroid hormone stores are depleted and the body can no longer compensate for the damage that is being done by the immune system. The body then settles into a hypothyroid state.

Because Hashimoto's can reflect either hypo- or hyper-thyroid states in the early stages, it can be associated with either anxiety or depression, depending on what is taking place in the body.

The HPT Axis – Case Studies

Checking for an underlying autoimmune process requires testing for specific thyroid antibodies, two of which are anti-thyroperoxidase (anti-TPO) and anti-thyroglobulin (anti-TG). Because the thyroid antibodies can cause symptoms before the TSH is even affected, it's possible for you to miss an underlying autoimmune process if your screening for thyroid dysfunction is limited to a TSH test.

For example, my teenage patient, Gracelynn, came to me with a concern of extreme fatigue that was affecting her performance at school; she had no other concerns at the time. In searching for the cause of her fatigue, I chose to evaluate her thyroid function. I checked her TSH, her thyroid hormones free T3 and free T4, and her thyroid antibodies, anti-TPO and anti-TG. When I received Gracelynn's lab results, her TSH was within the normal range at 0.936 uIU/ml (reference: 0.450-4.500 uIU/ml) and her anti-TG antibodies were high at 3.2 IU/ml (reference: 0.0-0.9). I ended up doing an additional test to rule out another autoimmune thyroid disorder, Grave's disease, but, at the end of the day, I had discovered the source of Gracelynn's fatigue—an underlying autoimmune thyroid disorder, Hashimoto's thyroiditis.

Because Gracelynn's Hashimoto's was still in its early stages, her TSH had not yet been significantly affected and was still within the normal range. Had I only run a TSH to screen for a thyroid disorder, I would have missed the cause of her fatigue and I would have also missed the opportunity to address the autoimmunity before it had the opportunity to progress. This is the main reason why I choose to do a more comprehensive thyroid panel when checking for thyroid disorders, instead of only checking TSH like most doctors do.

Now, here is the case of another patient, Monica, who presented with concerns of depression:

Monica was a 39-year-old female who reported persistent depression for the past several years. Before coming to me, she had been diagnosed with vitamin D deficiency for which she was prescribed high-dose vitamin D. This helped her mood somewhat, but her depression persisted. After talking with Monica, I found that she had been experiencing symptoms such as fatigue, difficulty losing weight despite a healthy diet, and excessive hair loss.

This alerted me to the fact that Monica's thyroid function may have been a contributing factor in her depression. We evaluated Monica's thyroid function and found that while her thyroid hormones were within the normal range, her TSH was just under 5 uIU/ml, which is much higher than where I like to see it. She also tested positive for anti-TPO and anti-TG antibodies outside of the normal range.

Having discovered that Hashimoto's was the cause of Monica's depression, I knew how to address it. I made lifestyle recommendations, recommendations to decrease Monica's thyroid antibodies, and botanical recommendations to support Monica's thyroid and adrenal glands. When Monica was able to follow up with me two months later, she had experienced a dramatic change. She reported a significant decrease in her hair loss and an improvement in her energy levels and in her mood. Monica reported laughing a few times within the weeks prior to her follow-up appointment, whereas she could not remember the last time she actually felt happy enough to laugh before then. I wish I could tell you that Monica's case is rare, but this is actually a very common occurrence.

Just as our HPG and HPT axes can significantly impact our mental health, our pathways for other hormones and neurotransmitters can also have a significant impact on our physical and mental wellbeing. This is why I take a comprehensive look into my patients' biological pathways when searching for causative and contributing factors to their mental states.

CHAPTER SIX

Profiles

· · · · · · · · · · · · · · · · · ·

When Profiling Goes Right

I N ADDRESSING THE THIRD P in the P7 Protocol™, *Profiles*, I analyze a variety of different factors that are unique to each individual in order to draw conclusions about their current state of health. This enables me to uncover specific problem areas that may be causing or contributing to poor mental health. Depending on the patient's history and symptoms, my profiling may include microbiome profiling, inflammatory marker profiling, environmental exposure profiling, or looking at other factors that can negatively impact mental health.

Gastrointestinal and Microbiome Profiling

Within the first few days of life, our gastrointestinal tracts are colonized by bacteria and other microbes. These microbes, when discussed as a whole, are referred to as the microbiome or the microbiota. Each microbe does something different within the body. Some have beneficial effects; some have little effect; others are beneficial under normal circumstances but can become harmful under specific conditions; and still others have dramatic, unrelenting negative effects on the body.

You may have heard about the gut-brain connection. Well, we now know that the microbes that colonize our gastrointestinal tracts are important to the function of the central nervous system and are able to influence the brain and its functions. Preclinical studies have shown that stressful events in the first few days and months of life, such as a traumatic birth or being separated from your mother, may change the composition and diversity of the microbiome even into adulthood.[20]

To further illustrate the effect of stress on the gastrointestinal system, I want you to think about the intestinal barrier, which prevents digesting food from passing directly into the bloodstream, as a sieve. When functioning optimally, this barrier allows certain particles to pass directly into the bloodstream, but prevents other particles from going through.

Before I explain more about the intestinal barrier, here's some important background information: the gastrointestinal system works very closely with the nervous system and the immune system. In fact, significant portions of the nervous and immune systems are actually housed within the gastrointestinal tract. The human enteric nervous system (what we call the network of nerve cells that are found in the gastrointestinal tract) contains between 200 and 600 million neurons.[21] For perspective, a cat's brain contains about 250 million neurons and a dog's brain contains about 500 million neurons.[22] The enteric nervous system communicates with the immune system, about 70% of which is housed in the gastrointestinal tract as gut-associated lymphoid tissue,[23] and the two work together to ward off invaders and accomplish other related functions.

Now, that we've discussed the relationships that exist between the gastrointestinal, nervous, and immune systems, let's revisit the subject of the intestinal barrier. A variety of factors, including changes in the microbiome, alcohol consumption, and consumption of the calorie-dense foods found in the standard American diet, all increase the permeability of the intestinal barrier.[24] This means that they widen the holes in the sieve I described earlier and allow easier passage of substances out of the gastrointestinal tract.

Stress is also an important factor that can increase the permeability of the gastrointestinal barrier. In the presence of stress, some microbes are also able to move more freely from one part of the gastrointestinal tract to another and to interact with the immune and nervous systems, affecting mental health.[20]

Researchers found that microbes are able to communicate with the brain via the immune system and via the enteric nervous system, and that this communication influences the HPA axis. These microbes' communication with the immune and nervous systems results in a hyper-reactive state, where the body sort of overreacts to higher stress levels. This then results in maladaptation to stress and varying degrees of depression in the long term.

This cascade of events begins with stressful events during the newborn period, which results in changes to the diversity and composition of the microbes of the gastrointestinal tract.[20]

In addition to affecting the brain indirectly by their effects on the immune and enteric nervous system, research shows that gut bacteria can also affect the brain directly. The vagus nerve, one of the 12 pairs of nerves that arise directly from the brain (as opposed to emerging from the spinal cord), plays a crucial role in the interconnectedness of the gut, the immune system, and the nervous system, including the brain. This nerve controls and communicates with the immune and nervous systems and it oversees digestion, immune response, and mood control.[25] Research shows that gut bacteria can impact brain function by influencing the activity of the vagus nerve.[26] This has implications in anxiety, depression, post-traumatic stress disorder, and other mental health concerns.

In addition to affecting mental health by communicating directly and indirectly with the brain, our microbiome can influence mental health in other ways. Many of our neurotransmitters (chemical messengers that are released at the end of nerve cells in order to facilitate communication and enact changes within the body) are produced by bacteria in the gut. Here are a few examples: we know that the Lactobacillus species produce acetylcholine and gamma-amino butyrate (GABA); the Bifidobacterium species also produce GABA; Escherichia species produce norepinephrine, serotonin, and dopamine; Streptococcus and Enterococcus species also produce serotonin; and Bacillus species produce dopamine and norepinephrine.[27] Abnormal concentrations of these neurotransmitters can contribute to or result in mood disorders and other mental health conditions.

You may be wondering, "If the microbiome has such significant effects on brain function and on mental health, and if changes in the composition of microbes in the gut relative to the microbes that are typically found in healthy individuals (referred to as dysbiosis or dysbiotic flora) lead to so many mental health concerns, then why can't we just adjust the microbiome in order to address the cause of these concerns?"

If that is your thought, you're definitely on to something. While the microbiome is a dynamic entity, influenced by several factors, including genetics, diet, metabolism, age, geography, antibiotic treatment, and stress, the evidence does suggest that influencing the gastrointestinal microbiome through targeted administration of certain strains of bacteria (especially specific strains of probiotics from the *Lactobacillus* and *Bifidobacterium* genera during the neonatal period and even later on in adulthood decreases hyper-reactivity of the HPA axis, promotes a more normal stress response, and improves mental health.[20,28]

GI and Microbiome Profiling – Case Study

Because gastrointestinal health is so closely connected to mental health, I take a comprehensive look at the bacteria and other microbes that are in my patients' gastrointestinal tracts. I also run tests to gather information about the level of inflammation present in the gastrointestinal tract and about the quality of digestion. This includes checking each patient's microbiome profile, looking at markers of inflammation such as fecal secretory IgA (SIgA) and calprotectin, looking at digestive enzymes and by-products of digestion, and more.

When I examine gastrointestinal profiles, one of the first things I check for is microbial diversity in the gut. A lack of microbial diversity is associated with many chronic physical and mental health conditions,[29] so I like to make sure that my patients have many different strains of beneficial bacteria and that the beneficial bacteria have what they need in order to proliferate and thrive.

After examining the makeup of the microbiome, I like to check for markers of inflammation. Fecal SIgA tends to be elevated either when the immune system in the gut is fighting opportunistic or otherwise harmful bacteria, yeast, parasites, or viruses in the gut or when the body is mounting an inflammatory response to food that the person is eating (e.g. food sensitivities). Another way that I gauge the inflammation level of the gastrointestinal tract is by looking at fecal calprotectin. Calprotectin, a protein that is released by cells under inflammatory conditions, is also a marker of gastrointestinal inflammation; what we've found is that the more inflamed the gastrointestinal tract is, the more calprotectin we see in stool samples.[30,31]

I also check pancreatic function in order to ensure that the enzymes that help digest macronutrients like fats and proteins are being produced and functioning appropriately. In addition to checking enzymes, I check for undigested components of these macronutrients in stool, which is another means of verifying that the pancreas is producing sufficient amounts of enzymes; if the pancreas isn't producing enough enzymes, then the food isn't fully digested, absorbed, and utilized, and we see undigested fats and proteins in the stool.

Now that I've shared some of the reasoning behind me taking such a comprehensive look into my patients' gastrointestinal health, I'll share a case study from one of my patients. Here's the example of one of my most recent patients, Shirley:

Shirley is a 49-year-old female who came to me with intense anxiety and associated tachycardia (increased heart rate), among other concerns. Shirley went in for a cardiology evaluation, which showed normal cardiac function on EKG. She also wore a heart monitor for 24 hours and the cardiologist did not find anything concerning.

The first time Shirley had experienced anything like these symptoms was after a round of antibiotics. She was also going through a stressful divorce at that time. Since then, she had been experiencing anxiety and tachycardia in response to eating certain foods (usually dairy) and in response to stressful situations. Shirley also reported severe bloating and told me that her anxiety and tachycardia improved after belching. Shirley reported seeing undigested food, such as rice and seeds, in her stool, indicating that she was not digesting her food well.

By the time she came to me, Shirley was plagued by daily anxiety, literally from a few moments after she woke up to when she closed her eyes at night. Her sleep was sometimes interrupted by anxious thoughts and tachycardia, and she feared going to sleep because she knew the cycle would repeat itself when she woke up the following morning.

While listening to Shirley's story, I was convinced that there was a gastrointestinal component to her anxiety. The fact that her cardiology evaluation results were all within normal limits, the fact that her first experience with these symptoms was after a round of antibiotics, the fact that she was extremely bloated and that releasing some of that gas led to improvements in her anxiety and tachycardia, and even the fact that she said her body was "no longer responding well to stress" (which suggests HPA axis dysregulation) all screamed gastrointestinal crisis and dysbiotic flora to me.

Shirley's gastrointestinal health evaluation confirmed my suspicions. Her test results revealed microbial imbalance including high levels of potentially pathogenic bacteria, low levels of some strains of beneficial bacteria, and abnormally high levels of bacteria that are normally found in the gastrointestinal tract. For example, her levels of *Escherichia coli*, a strain of bacteria that is normally found in the gut, were double the upper limit of what's considered normal. *Escherichia* bacteria can slow the rate at which food travels through the gastrointestinal tract, leading to an imbalance in the gastrointestinal flora.[32] *Escherichia coli* can also produce a signaling molecule called indole, and research suggests that individuals whose gut bacteria are highly prone to producing indole are at increased risk of developing anxiety and other mood disorders because of the molecule's ability to activate and influence the vagus nerve.[33]

There was also a very high amount of *Citrobacter* bacteria present. *Citrobacter*, another genus that is normally found in the gastrointestinal tract, produces gas and bloating in the gut as a by-product of its glucose fermentation process.[34] *Citrobacter* can be harmful under specific circumstances and, although we haven't noted this effect in humans, we do know that the presence of some strains has been associated with anxiety-like behaviors in preclinical models.[35] In the research, these anxiety-like behaviors did not come about as a result of the bacteria's effect on gastrointestinal inflammation or gut health in general; instead, evidence suggests that these behaviors came about as a direct result of the bacteria's effect on and communication with the vagus nerve.[35]

Shirley's results also showed abnormally elevated fecal SIgA and she had by-products of protein digestion in her stool, indicating that her digestive enzymes were not able to fully digest her food and that her body was not able to fully absorb the food that she was eating. Additionally, her levels of *Akkermansia muciniphila*, a specific strain of bacteria that releases enzymes that regulate the buildup of the mucosal layer and consequently strengthens the gut barrier, were below the detectable limit.[36]

Suffice it to say that Shirley had a lot going on in her gastrointestinal tract that was contributing to and possibly even directly causing her anxiety. By the time she came to me, she had been to 4 different practitioners, she was on more than 12 different supplements, and she had been on quite a few different medications as well. Some of the supplements that she was taking were high-quality, professional-grade supplements that I use in my own practice, but because of the way that they were used, they were actually hindering her healing.

For example, Shirley was on a gut-healing supplement that contained polysaccharides and other prebiotics. You can think of prebiotics as food for bacteria. Supplementing prebiotics along with probiotics helps to ensure that the bacteria have what they need in order to survive and actually colonize the gut. At first glance, prebiotics may seem like a great idea for Shirley, and they would be if they were taken at the appropriate time. This, however, wasn't the time.

In addition to feeding beneficial bacteria such as *Lactobacillus* and *Bifidobacterium* strains, prebiotics can also feed potentially harmful bacteria,[37] causing them to further multiply and occupy even more of the gastrointestinal tract. In patients experiencing severe gastrointestinal symptoms, it's important to ensure that there isn't any bacterial overgrowth taking place in the small or large intestines and that the ratios and strains of bacteria in the gut are reasonably close to optimal before administering prebiotics; if this isn't the case and you supplement with prebiotics, you'll likely experience a worsening of your gastrointestinal symptoms.

Because Shirley did have abnormal concentrations of many strains of bacteria, a more appropriate course of action for her would have been to:

1. Change her diet to include foods that are most conducive to the growth and development of healthy gut flora and exclude those that aren't.

2. Use antimicrobial agents to address dysbiosis by eradicating potentially pathogenic bacteria and other microbes and supporting the return of her beneficial gastrointestinal flora to more normal concentrations.

3. Support her body's digestion and absorption by supplementing with appropriate digestive enzymes in order to decrease her gas and bloating and ensure that she absorbs her nutrients appropriately.

4. Once dysbiotic flora is eradicated, re-inoculate the gastrointestinal tract with probiotics and supplement with prebiotics as well in order to help the probiotics to colonize the gut and proliferate.

5. Provide the gastrointestinal tract with the key nutrients that are necessary for its rebuilding and repair.

I developed and discussed this long-term plan with
Shirley and then made specific recommendations to start.
I had Shirley discontinue her prebiotic-containing supplements as well as two other supplements that I believed
were causing more harm than good. I made dietary recommendations, I had her discontinue or continue until she
finished six other supplements (I didn't feel that they were
necessary and I really wanted to consolidate her treatment
plan to include only a few hard-hitting supplements and/
or therapies), I started her on some antimicrobial agents to
begin the process of eradicating the potentially pathogenic
bacteria, and I had her continue the digestive enzymes that
she had been taking in order to begin our first phase of her
gut-healing protocol. I also made other recommendations
to address her chronic, physical health concerns.

While we worked at addressing the cause of her anxiety
by optimizing her gastrointestinal system and her physical health concerns, I made recommendations to acutely
address Shirley's anxiety by supporting her body's production of calming neurotransmitters like GABA. Addressing
all of Shirley's physical and mental health concerns will
take a few months, but when we last spoke (about 5 weeks
into implementing the first phase of her treatment plan),

she reported that her anxiety had significantly decreased and she sounded much less anxious than she did at our initial meeting.

In addition to looking at gastrointestinal health and the microbiome when evaluating my patients' profiles, I may also conduct environmental exposure profiling in order to evaluate for heavy metal or chemical exposures that can contribute to mental health conditions, inflammatory marker profiling in order to evaluate the effect that inflammation is having on mental health, or biotoxin or other biological agent profiling to evaluate the hidden roles that mold exposure or other biologic exposure may be playing in my patients' poor mental health.

CHAPTER SEVEN

Personalization

. . . .

Unique Body Seeks Unique Treatment

WHEN ADDRESSING *PERSONALIZATION*, THE fourth P in the P7 Protocol™, I consider my patients' current state of health including their diagnosed conditions and other symptoms as well as their lifestyle habits. Once I have a good understanding of these factors, I make appropriate recommendations to help them adopt the most health-producing lifestyle possible given each of their unique circumstances.

Elimination & Challenge Protocol

In my 6-month program, I usually begin addressing diet by having my patients go through my elimination and challenge protocol where they eliminate all inflammatory foods and the most common food sensitivities for

3 to 4 weeks. At the end of that time period, my patients reintroduce some previously eliminated foods back into their diets one at a time by eating that specific food at each meal on a given day.

When testing foods for reintroduction, I always instruct people to test them in their purest forms. As an example, you wouldn't test wheat by eating a pepperoni pizza. If you are testing wheat, then you want to be sure that any return of symptoms is due to the wheat itself and not to the tomato sauce, the pepperoni, the cheese, or anything else on the pizza. The way to be sure is to keep everything else in your diet constant and ensure that the only new variable being added to your diet at that time is the wheat. In this way, you'll be better able to definitively attribute any return of symptoms that you experience to the reintroduction of wheat into your diet.

It's important to pay close attention to changes in your mood and other relevant symptoms that you experience while reintroducing foods into your diet. During reintroduction, I have my patients keep a daily log of their symptoms so that we can accurately track their symptoms. If a patient isn't sure if they've reacted negatively to a food,

I have them retest in 4-5 days. If a patient's symptoms worsen after reintroducing a specific food, I have them completely eliminate that food from their diet for 6-12 months before attempting to retest.

While I have done and still do food sensitivity testing for some patients under very specific circumstances, I've found the elimination and challenge protocol to be the most effective means of identifying food sensitivities and constructing a personalized diet plan for my patients.

Time Spent In Nature Versus In Urban Areas

When it comes to lifestyle interventions, one of my favorite interventions to recommend to my patients is that they spend time in a natural environment as often as possible. This is because exposure to "green space" such as forests and parks has been positively associated with mental health benefits such as decreased stress; decreased mental fatigue; reductions in crime, violence, and aggression; decreased incidences of chronic disease; and better overall health[38]. Regardless of the type of community that you live in, your socioeconomic status, your age, your marital status, and other potentially confounding factors, the presence of green space in your neighborhood is associated with lower levels of depression, anxiety, and stress and improved mental health outcomes.[38]

If your actual neighborhood doesn't have much green space, but there are parks in the vicinity, you can still experience the benefits of green space exposure. Research shows that the closer you live to green space, the better it is for your overall health. Compared to people in neighborhoods where the closest green space was 3 kilometers away, people living in neighborhoods that were 1 kilometer away from green space had significantly lower levels of anxiety, depression, and medically unexplained physical symptoms.[39] This study was significant because researchers had conducted similar research by asking participants about their health (e.g. self-reported symptoms), which leaves some room for error, but the data from this study actually came specifically from the medical records of 195 primary care physicians, indicating that these results were based on cases of medically-observable, diagnosed health conditions rather than on participants' reports.

While the presence of green space is associated with improved mental health outcomes, the opposite is true as well. The absence of green space is associated with poor mental health outcomes. For example, for individuals experiencing psychosis, spending time in urban environments led to increased negative thoughts about other people, increased paranoia, and increased anxiety.[40] For those experiencing delusions, spending time in busy urban areas led to significant increases in paranoia, hearing voices, anxiety, negative beliefs about oneself, and negative beliefs about others.[41]

I recommend that my patients spend some time in green space each week or as often as possible, even if it is simply sitting or walking in their back yards, because of its proven benefits for mental and overall wellbeing.

Physical Activity

Engaging in physical activity can also have a profound positive impact on mental health. We believe this may be due to the release of beta-endorphins after exercise. When we exercise or are otherwise physically active, our bodies release chemicals called endorphins. Endorphins are endogenous opioid neuropeptides, meaning that they are produced within the body and act on opioid receptors, similar to the synthetic opiate drugs that we're familiar with such as morphine and hydrocodone. When we engage in physical activity, endorphins interact with our brains to decrease anxiety, depression, and our perception of pain.

Physical activity reduces anxiety and improves feelings of wellbeing. It has also been shown to be as effective as anti-depressant medication in the treatment of mild to moderate depression, and it has been shown to improve mood when used in conjunction with medication in the treatment of severe depression.[42]

In addition to being beneficial in cases of anxiety and depression, physical activity is beneficial for people who are at risk for schizophrenia and those experiencing psychosis. It improves physical health and helps to reduce risk factors for schizophrenia such as metabolic dysregulation.

Brain-derived neurotrophic factor (BDNF) is a protein that plays a major role in the survival, growth, maturation, and maintenance of brain and nerve cells. Because it stimulates neuroplasticity by promoting the expression of BDNF, physical activity enhances the brain's ability to form new connections and our ability to learn new behaviors and thoughts.[43] The increased expression of BDNF, which comes about as a result of physical activity promotes neurogenesis, which makes physical activity an effective means of aiding the body in restoring areas of the brain that are damaged during psychotic episodes.[44]

Moderate-intensity exercise has been shown to improve both positive and negative symptoms of schizophrenia as well as cognitive and functional abilities.[44]

Because of the many benefits of physical activity on mental health, I help my patients incorporate patterns of healthy movement throughout their days and develop personalized exercise plans, both of which help them secure the benefits associated with physical activity in a way that is feasible, practical, and as compatible with their lifestyles as possible.

Nature-Based Activities

If you're not the type of person who likes structured exercise in a gym or a group class, you can still secure the mental health benefits associated with physical activity by spending time engaged in nature-based activities like hiking and walking on trails. In fact, the mental health benefits that are associated with exercise increase when the physical activity takes place in nature, so you actually have the potential to experience more of the benefits.

Research shows that engaging in physical activity while in green space leads to significant reduction in anxiety symptoms for people diagnosed with anxiety;[45] feelings of improved mood for individuals diagnosed with major depressive disorder and bipolar type II;[46] and decreased anxiety, decreased stress levels, and an increased sense of calmness for individuals diagnosed with post-traumatic stress disorder.[47]

Walking in a rural environment was associated with improvements in mood, general positive feelings, and feelings of vitality and restoration. Negative feelings such as tension, anxiety, depression and confusion decreased while walking in this environment.[48]

When engaging in physical activity, doing so in a natural environment is preferable to doing so in a facility or institution; however, if that isn't a possibility, it's important to remember that any physical activity is preferable to no physical activity at all.

The Importance of Sleep

There is a very strong connection between sleep and mental health and the link is inflammation. Poor sleep quality leads to an increase in inflammation, which negatively impacts the development and course of mental health concerns. When a person is completely sleep-deprived, such as if he or she does not sleep at all for two or more nights, we see an increase in c-reactive protein (CRP), a commonly-tested marker for inflammation within the body. If, instead of being totally sleep-deprived, a person is partially sleep-deprived—such as if he or she gets sub-optimal quantities or quality of sleep for a longer period of time—we see an increase in interleukin-6, a pro-inflammatory marker that is produced in the body whenever there is acute or chronic inflammation.

Increased levels of interleukin-6 are associated with major depression, bipolar disorder, and other affective disorders.[49] Essentially, sleep disturbances lead to an increase in interleukin-6, which leads to the onset or worsening of mental health concerns, which then leads to an increase in sleep disturbances, and the cycle continues.

Similarly, lack of sleep increases a person's risk of developing eating disorders such as anorexia nervosa, bulimia nervosa, binge-eating disorder, and nighttime eating syndrome, while having an eating disorder increases the likelihood of having an increase in sleep disturbances. In addition to these relationships, lack of sleep has been associated with greater symptom severity and impaired daytime functioning in individuals with eating disorders.[50] Disturbed sleep is also associated with increased severity of anxiety and irritability.[51,52]

Sleep and immunological processes also play a significant role in schizophrenia. Between 30 and 80% of people diagnosed with schizophrenia report sleep disturbances. Research shows increases in pro-inflammatory cytokines such as interleukin-6, interleukin-10, and TNF-alpha in individuals with schizophrenia as well, indicating that these sleep disturbances may be related to changes in inflammation levels.[49]

Because of these crucial connections between sleep, inflammation, and mental health, I recommend that my patients aim for 7-8 hours of sleep each night; and for my patients with insomnia, I may make recommendations to regulate their circadian rhythm (internal clocks), address any anxiety or discomfort that may be preventing them from sleeping, or induce sleep at the appropriate time in order to help them achieve this goal.

During the *Personalization* portion of the P7 Protocol™, I assess and address my patients' diet in order to lay the foundation for health, and we adjust beverage consumption, time spent in nature, level of physical activity, and sleep quality. Through health coaching and setting specific, achievable lifestyle goals, we help our patients construct a comprehensive lifestyle plan that lays the foundation for health within the body and gets them on the fast-track to progress along their own individual healing journey.

CHAPTER EIGHT

Panoptic Inventory

. . . .

A Broad View For a New You

W HEN ADDRESSING THE FIFTH P, I help my patients
take a *Panoptic Inventory* of their lives. Through this
panoptic inventory, we take a comprehensive look at how
each aspect of humanity—physical, mental, spiritual, and
social—influences the others, so that we can identify any
roadblocks that may be hindering their progress along their
wellness journeys.

When addressing mental health in a clinical setting, it's a
given that your doctor, psychiatrist, or therapist will address
the mental and emotional aspects. If you're working with
a doctor who is seeking to address the underlying cause,
you'll likely address components of physical health as well,
but it's very seldom that we address the other aspects of

our being—the social and spiritual aspects—and yet these two areas are so intimately connected to mental and physical wellness and can be such powerful vehicles to help us progress along our wellness journeys.

As humans, we are all social beings, and the social aspects of humanity have significant effects on mental wellness. In fact, individuals with strong social support systems and a strong sense of community enjoy better mental health compared to those who do not have these things.[53] Additionally, research demonstrates that regardless of the level of social support individuals actually receive, if they perceive that they have high levels of social support, then they are less likely to suffer adverse physiological complications from their diagnosed health conditions.[54]

Spirituality has a significant effect on mental health as well and can be a powerful driving force on the journey of recovery. It's also possible for our experiences with religion and spirituality to negatively impact our mental health. Whether they have a positive or negative impact on mental health depends largely on our past experiences and the types of coping strategies we employ.

When coping with life stressors and mental health concerns we can choose to employ either positive coping strategies, such as prayer, meditation, and a healthy spiritual outlook, or we can choose to employ negative coping strategies, which would involve a more negative spiritual outlook.

In a study regarding spiritual coping strategies, researchers had participants complete a survey by selecting how often they resorted to a variety of different coping strategies. The survey included a list of positive religious coping strategies such as "Looked for a stronger connection with God" and "Tried to see how God might be trying to strengthen me in this situation," and negative religious coping strategies such as "Wondered what I did for God to punish me" and "Questioned God's love for me." Survey choices included "Not at all," "Somewhat," "Quite a bit," and "A great deal."[55]

At the end of the study, research demonstrated that those who employed positive religious coping strategies had lower levels of depression compared to those who did not. Those using these positive coping methods were also more likely to report better quality and perception of life, shortened length of hospitalization, decreased mortality, improved immune function, and better overall health and vitality.[55]

A similar study found that higher levels of religion or spirituality may help buffer risk for mental health disorders including post-traumatic stress disorder, major depressive disorder, alcohol abuse disorder, and suicidal ideation.[56]

While positive religious coping has been strongly associated with better health outcomes, negative coping strategies can also have negative effects on mental health. For example, research shows that people who employ negative spiritual coping strategies such as believing that they've been abandoned or are being punished by God, feeling guilty or ashamed, and questioning God's power or love, are at an increased risk of being diagnosed with one or more mental health condition(s). They're also more likely to experience more severe symptoms than those who don't employ negative coping strategies.[57]

To summarize, here we have a situation where those who employ negative coping strategies are at increased risk of being diagnosed with mental health conditions and experiencing more severe symptoms compared to those who do not utilize any spiritual coping strategies, positive or negative, and those who utilize positive coping strategies. At the same time, those who utilize positive spiritual coping strategies and have higher levels of religion or spirituality are at the greatest advantage, because they are much less likely to be diagnosed with mental health conditions and, in the event that they are diagnosed with one or more mental health conditions, their symptoms tend to be less severe than the other two groups we've discussed.

Understanding the benefit that positive coping strategies and religion/spirituality have on mental health, we should be asking questions like, "What is the source or origin of negative coping strategies?" and "How can we help individuals with negative or no coping strategies to develop positive coping strategies?"

Here's what I've found: In my experience, the tendency to utilize negative spiritual coping strategies stems from our personal experiences in early life. For example, if a woman is raised in a religion or environment that views God as demanding and tyrannical, then it will only be natural for her to feel that the negative circumstances she is undergoing are a direct result of her being punished by God or for her to resort to other forms of negative coping.

Here's another hypothetical example: most Christian denominations describe God as a loving and caring Father. If a man's father abused him, you can see how it might be difficult for him to view God as a Father while at the same time believing that God is loving and caring; he has no frame of reference from which to make such a comparison. Having never experienced a father's love and care, he may have subconsciously come to the conclusion that fathers are not loving, don't truly care about their children, and actually want to see them being hurt by circumstances and by life.

And finally, here's a quick real-life example: my patient Carol had been diagnosed with bipolar disorder type I. Carol had been raised in a dysfunctional household; she was physically and sexually abused as a child. Her family espoused the Christian faith, but they did not go to church very often. As can be expected, Carol did learn some things from her family members about God and religion that had negatively impacted the way she experienced Christianity. She started to adopt negative coping strategies from an early age, and by the time she came to me, she reported feeling condemned with a heavy weight of guilt. She felt that God was upset with and disappointed in her, and this belief was serving as a major barrier to her healing. I did have the opportunity to talk with Carol about these false beliefs that she had adopted, and she acknowledged that they were both false and serving as a barrier, which, of course, is the first step in overcoming the negative effects that these types of coping strategies can have on mental health.

Because utilizing negative coping skills can have negative effects on mental health and hinder your progress along your wellness journey, taking a spiritual and emotional inventory that assesses your coping strategies and considers the emotions that are associated with them and their origin can be of great benefit. If you are in the habit of utilizing negative coping strategies, then realizing this fact is the first step toward making a change. Transitioning to a place where you are comfortably using more positive coping strategies (and experiencing the improved mental wellbeing and better health outcomes that come along with positive coping) is the next step on the path to using spirituality, belief, and hope to your advantage along your mental wellness journey.

CHAPTER NINE

Professionals

· · · · · · · · · · · · · · · · ·

Teamwork Makes the Dream Work

W HEN ADDRESSING THE SIXTH P, *Professionals*, we encourage our patients to work with relevant professionals who are a good fit for them. This ensures that each patient has the collaborative medical team that he or she needs in order to successfully regain optimal mental wellness. The professionals that we recommend that our patients work with could include psychiatrists and other prescribing clinicians, therapists or counselors, licensed massage therapists, colon hydrotherapists, neurofeedback technicians, health coaches, or other relevant professionals.

In my experience, every professional is not the ideal fit for every patient. For example, research shows that cognitive behavioral therapy activities such as self-monitoring and cognitive restructuring can be extremely beneficial in helping to address mood disorders and other mental health concerns.[58] Because of this, when I believe it will be of benefit, I recommend that my patients work with a knowledgeable cognitive behavioral therapist who can help them address habits such as negative self-talk using those and similar activities. In spite of what the research shows, some of my patients have reported that cognitive behavioral therapy has not been helpful for them. Curious as to why, I decided to look further into the matter. What I found was that most, if not all, of my patients who reported not benefitting from cognitive behavioral therapy also reported that they were never really able to connect with their therapists on a personal level or they didn't quite resonate with the therapists' style or approach to therapy. In other words, the issue wasn't so much with the therapy as it was with the therapist.

Understanding this, we encourage our patients to work with professionals who are a good fit for them and we make recommendations for these professionals whenever indicated and possible. While working with our patients to restore mental wellness, I've found providing additional support by means of other professionals to be an important factor in many of my patients' outcomes.

After reading this book, it's only natural for you to attempt to implement the concepts you've learned into your daily life in an attempt to improve your own mental health. In doing so, I recommend that you work with your primary care physician and/or other members of your medical team. I highly recommend that you reach out to relevant professionals for help when you need it and that you search for practitioners who are the best fit for you and whose philosophies of healing align with your own. I truly believe that doing so will expedite your healing process.

CHAPTER TEN

Prescriptions

· · · · · · · · · · · · · · · · · ·

Do You Ever Need Medication?

W HEN ADDRESSING THE SEVENTH and final P, *Pre-scriptions*, I explain to my patients the role that psychiatric medication should play in restoring mental wellness and I assist my patients with either tapering off their medications or integrating them with their naturopathic care.

All medication that is legally distributed in the United States, including medication that is prescribed to address psychiatric concerns, is regulated by the United States Food and Drug Administration (FDA). The FDA is the official regulatory body for pharmaceutical medication in this country, but the fact that the FDA approves a drug does not necessarily mean that we know and understand the implications of its use or all of the short- and long-term effects of the drug. Oftentimes it takes several years, more than thirty in some cases, for the unintended effects of a drug to command enough attention to necessitate the FDA stepping in and legislating the appropriate level of change.

Here's a common scenario: a drug is FDA-approved and practitioners begin to prescribe the drug for its intended use. After 10, 20, or more years of prescribing the drug, it becomes undeniably clear that its use is associated with some unwanted effect, such as liver failure or an increase in suicidal ideation. The FDA then insists that manufacturers of the drug place a black-box warning (the strictest warning that the FDA requires to be placed in the labeling of drugs when there is reasonable evidence that their use is associated with a serious hazard) or some other warning on the drug label, or they ban the sale and administration of the drug completely within the United States.

My purpose in sharing that scenario was to illustrate the fact that our understanding of psychiatric medications and their effects on the brain and body is continually evolving. In the case of some drugs, such as *Seroquel* (quetiapine fumarate),[59] which is prescribed in cases of schizophrenia and in cases of mania as seen in bipolar disorder, we are still unclear about exactly how they work. It would be absurd for us to pretend that we currently understand all that there is to be understood about the short- and long-term effects of these drugs.

We do know that each drug initially has a specific effect on the individual. For example, the serotonin-specific reuptake inhibitor *Zoloft* (sertraline) blocks the uptake of serotonin, allowing more of the neurotransmitter to remain in the synapse for longer periods of time. Over time, however, the brain begins to make its own adjustments, and it compensates for the drug's initial effect. In the case of *Zoloft*, research shows that the chronic administration of this drug leads to the down-regulation of the brain's receptors for norepinephrine, another neurotransmitter.[60]

As illustrated in this example, when we factor in the brain's own compensatory mechanisms which take place over time, we find that it's no longer a case of "Zoloft and the other SSRIs work by affecting the serotonin pathway," but instead, the effect of psychotropic drugs becomes even more complicated than we once believed. When we add in additional variables by prescribing multiple drugs concurrently, the effects of these drugs become even less predictable.

The Role Of Psychiatric Medication

My understanding of these facts as well as my training in and experience with pharmaceutical medications have significantly impacted my philosophy of healing, specifically as it pertains to the administration of psychiatric medication. My philosophy of healing regarding psychotropic medication is this: I believe that medication plays an important role in addressing acute psychiatric concerns. I also believe that psychotropic medication should not be our long-term solution.

Here's an example of why I say the use of psychotropic medication should be limited to short-term use: research suggests that higher numbers of manic episodes in bipolar disorder may be associated with decreased frontal cortical volume.[61] To put it simply, the research suggests that manic episodes, such as are seen in bipolar and in schizophrenia, may result in brain shrinkage. Given this information, I believe it is important to address acute episodes of mania as quickly as possible, and pharmaceutical medications play a significant role in doing so.

At the same time, however, a significant body of research suggests that the long-term administration of all classes of psychotropic medication result in loss of brain mass and/or function, similar to that which is seen in other forms of trauma to the brain including sports-induced and other forms of traumatic brain injury and electroconvulsive therapy. This syndrome has come to be referred to in the literature as chronic brain impairment (CBI).[62]

CBI is characterized by four major groups of symptoms that, together, result is decreased quality of life.[62]

These symptoms include:

1. cognitive dysfunction including difficulty with short-term memory and learning new things, inattention, and poor concentration;

2. apathy, loss of energy and vitality, and fatigue;

3. emotional worsening, which includes loss of empathy, increased impatience and anger, and frequent mood changes;

4. and a lack of self-awareness of these symptoms (e.g. people other than the person who is taking the drug notice these symptoms, but the patient may have a difficult time seeing what others see).

While we don't want to leave any mental health concern unaddressed, we also don't want to limit ourselves and our attempts to address these concerns to pharmaceutical medication. I believe that every mental health concern warrants a formulaic, comprehensive, functional, and foundational approach that looks at and treats the whole person, not just their symptoms or their diagnosed conditions. My philosophy of healing involves seeking to identify the underlying causes of the concern and addressing them in the manner that maximizes effectiveness and minimizes long-term, negative effects. I stay up-do-date on the latest research, because I'm on a continual search to identify therapies and treatments that have safer and safer side-effect profiles and yet can effectively help my patients to obtain optimal mental wellness.

As we've discussed, the formulaic approach that I take involves laying the foundation for health by optimizing genetics and lifestyle, addressing biochemical and hormonal pathways that may be contributing to poor mental health, providing the body with what it needs in order to facilitate its return to a state of wellness, addressing past trauma and negative emotions that may serve as a barrier to healing, getting relevant professionals on board as needed to ensure that each patient has the collaborative medical team that he or she needs, and utilizing psychiatric medication when necessary, either in cases of acute need or in cases where their use can be helpful in the process of tapering off of medications that are stronger and more likely to induce chemical dependency.

Medication Tapering

Regarding the process of tapering off medications, I only initiate this process with my patients after we've laid the foundation for health, I've seen sufficient subjective and objective improvements in my patients' health, and the patient and I collaboratively decide that it is a good time to begin the process of discontinuing the medication.

The brain gradually compensates for the changes that drugs impose upon it, and abrupt removal of a drug does not allow the brain enough time to adjust to the changing concentrations of the drug. In most cases, this leads to unpleasant withdrawal symptoms. To limit these unwanted effects, I help my patients discontinue their medication using an incremental weaning protocol that takes into consideration factors such as how long the patient has been on the medication, the patient's current symptoms, genetics, and other factors that affect the rate at which a person can wean off of a medication. While weaning off of medication, I maintain close communication with my patients and support their moods as indicated using natural therapies. Many of my patients have been able to decrease their medication dosage or discontinue their medication altogether using this approach.

CHAPTER ELEVEN

I Eat; Therefore, I Think

· · · · · · · · · · · · · · · · · ·

How Food Choices Affect Mental Health

WITH ALL OF THE nutrition- and diet-related information available today, it's difficult to know exactly what route to take. What should you be eating in order to obtain and best maintain optimal mental health? What is the ideal diet for optimal wellness? Because I truly want you to understand how to navigate the information that's out there, I'll share my secret with you.

Here it is: whenever you are approaching a topic that is likely to have several different (and oftentimes opposing) points of view, it's important to look at the totality of evidence; you need to look at the research with a critical eye.

In other words, it is possible to prove almost any viewpoint using limited or skewed evidence. When you take a wider and deeper look, however, and assess all of the evidence available to you, you'll come out with a more balanced and well-rounded understanding of the subject.

You might ask, "Dr. Louis, if it's so simple, then why doesn't everyone take this approach?"

I have two reasons for you. Here they are:

1. This approach takes time and determination.
2. Food is big business.

I'll explain what I mean.

This Approach Takes Time & Determination

The fact that this approach takes time and determination is pretty straightforward. We can all agree that it's much easier to read or hear about a study or a concept and instantly become its greatest advocate and evangelist than it is to take the time to analyze the research, consider the opposing arguments, and then espouse a specific viewpoint.

The fact of the matter is that, in today's fast-paced world, very few people are motivated enough to consider the totality of evidence before jumping on a bandwagon. It takes a very special type of person, one who isn't easily deterred and who possesses an earnest desire for knowledge, truth, and, in this case, optimal health, to be willing to go through the oftentimes confusing research and draw an accurate conclusion.

Food Is Big Business

My second reason was that food is big business. If anyone desires to dispute this fact, I simply point them back to an April 1996 episode of The Oprah Winfrey Show. Do you remember? In April of '96, Oprah decided to discuss the mad cow disease outbreak and the related Creutzfeldt-Jakob Disease that had occurred in Great Britain with Howard Lyman, an organic farmer and animal rights activist. The practice of feeding processed livestock to cattle had been linked to the European outbreak, and Lyman criticized this act. In response to his statements, Oprah stated that he had "just stopped me cold from eating another burger."[63]

Two years after the show, the cattle ranchers in the beef industry decided to sue both Oprah Winfrey and Howard

Lyman, stating that Oprah's remarks had led to a dramatic decrease in the cost of beef, sending prices to a 10-year low and costing the industry $12 million dollars. They were seeking damages from the defendants in the amount of almost $11 million. The cattle ranchers were able to sue Winfrey and Lyman under a law that had been passed in Texas in 1995, the year prior to the show being aired.

At the time in the United States, similar laws existed in 13 other states. These laws essentially state that people can be held liable if they make false and disparaging claims about perishable food products. After a 5-week trial heard by 12 jurors, however, it was ruled in favor of the defendants, stating that they were only exercising their first amendment right to freedom of speech.[64]

This is only one example of food being big business. History and the present are filled with additional examples of people suing people for statements against their industries, of big industries sponsoring research that supports their cause and providing inducements to scientists and physicians in order to accomplish this goal, of big industries refusing to publish research after the results did not support their cause, of big businesses skewing research in order to make it appear as though it supports their cause, and much, much more. I don't say all this in order to convince you to become a conspiracy theorist, but rather to encourage you to have a second and a third look at the research you encounter and to look at it with a critical eye.

In order to critically and intelligently analyze the research, you need to first understand that there are varying levels of evidence when it comes to research. For example, the evidence gathered from a case study, which typically reports the experience of one person, would not be as strong as evidence gathered from a randomized controlled trial, which is a term used to describe a research setup where participants are divided into two or more groups and all variables but one (the therapy in question) are kept relatively constant among participants across the groups.

Randomized controlled trials usually include blinding, which increases their reliability. In a randomized, double-blind, controlled clinical trial, participants are randomly distributed into intervention and no-intervention groups and neither the experimenters nor the participants know which participants are receiving which therapy (or no therapy at all in the case of the no-intervention or control group). This helps to reduce the likelihood of any bias occurring either because of the experimenters' beliefs about what the outcome should be or because of the participants' expectations about how their health should be affected based on their knowledge about the therapies that they are or aren't receiving.

Types Of Research

As far as the level of evidence is concerned, here is a list of different study designs in research ordered from least reliable to most reliable when it comes to translating the conclusions of these studies to humans: [65]

1. Animal studies: studies done on animals are least reliable because results don't always transfer across species, but this is typically where we start when a person comes up with an idea for research.

2. Case study or case series: a case series consists of a collection of case studies on the treatment of individual patients while a case study is a report on a single patient. These can be more reliable than animal studies, but because they are reports of cases

and there aren't any control groups for comparison, they are still lower on the level of evidence ladder.

3. Case-control studies: case-control studies look back and compare people who have been diagnosed with a specific condition with people who do not have that condition. Researchers try to draw conclusions about factors that could have caused the condition. These are less reliable than cohort studies and randomized controlled trials because, in addition to medical records, they rely on people's ability to recall information after the fact for data collection and are therefore subject to recall bias. Additionally, the fact that there is an association between a given factor and the outcome (the disease) does not necessarily mean that the factor in question caused the outcome.

4. Cohort studies: cohort studies locate people who are already doing or taking a certain intervention and then follow them over time and compare their outcomes with a group of similar people who did not do or take that intervention. These studies are more reliable than case-control studies because they include a larger group of people, but they aren't as

reliable as randomized control trials since the two groups of people in cohort studies may differ by more variables than the one that's being studied.

5. Randomized controlled trials: as discussed, randomized controlled trials randomly divide participants into a control (no-intervention) group and one or more experimental (those receiving the intervention or treatment) groups. All variables but the treatment in question are kept constant. Blinding and randomization reduce the likelihood of bias in these studies, making randomized controlled trials the most reliable form of evidence used to evaluate the effectiveness of an intervention.

6. Systematic reviews: systematic reviews don't directly involve experimental research conducted on participants. Instead, researchers who conduct systematic reviews search the body of available research in an attempt to answer a specific question. They then summarize the most reliable research available pertaining to that question in order to construct a concluding response to the question. Because systematic reviews rely on the most reliable data, many of the inclusion

criteria for these studies stipulate that a study must be a randomized controlled trial to be included.

7. Meta-analyses: meta-analyses don't directly involve experimental research conducted on participants either. To conduct meta-analyses, researchers search the body of available research for the most reliable data and use mathematical equations to combine the data as though it were one large study in order to draw conclusions.

In addition to the study designs I mentioned, we can gather information through cross-sectional studies. Cross-sectional studies are a special type of study that shows the relationship between diseases and other factors in a pre-defined group of people at a specific point in time. They are different from the other studies because they do not follow people over a period of time; instead they look at a group of people and try to gather information about associations between diseases and other factors at a given point in time.

While cross-sectional studies can show associations, they don't provide any information about cause and effect. For example, a cross-sectional study may reveal an association between depression and nutritional deficiencies in a group of people, but it doesn't provide us with enough information to say whether the depression led to poor eating habits, which led to nutritional deficiencies; the nutritional deficiencies caused the depression; or if there is another causative agent involved.

Cohort, cross sectional, and case-control studies are all considered to be observational studies. Observational studies are generally viewed as being less reliable than randomized controlled trials because of the fact that the researchers have no control over the variables in observational studies.

Now that we're on the same page regarding the most relevant types of studies in order of reliability, let's get back to diet and mental health.

A Look At The Current Research

There's a reason why I dedicated the last several pages to explaining the difference between the various types of research and their levels of reliability to you. The fact is that there are many well-meaning people who teach that adhering to certain diets is the best way to address or reverse mental health concerns like depression and anxiety, but their reasoning is based on cohort studies that looked at only a small number of people and other less reliable research. As we now know, cohort studies aren't as reliable as randomized controlled trials because it's difficult to keep all variables but one constant in these types of studies.

In 2013, researchers wanted to find out what influence diet really had on mental health, specifically depression, so they conducted a systematic review and meta-analysis of all of the literature in six different electronic databases. The results of this review stated that high intakes of fruit, vegetables, fish, and whole grains may be associated with reduced mental health risk, but the conclusion came with the caveat that we need more high-quality randomized controlled trials and cohort studies in order to confirm these findings.[66]

The reason for the caveat was the fact that, of the 4502 studies initially identified, only 13 met the inclusion criteria, and, of those 13, only 1 study was a randomized controlled trial. The researchers noted that, although their study was the most comprehensive evaluation of the then-current research, most of the evidence was cross-sectional in nature, so while the research is useful in showing associations, it is limited in that it cannot determine whether poor diet caused poor mental health or poor mental health led to poor dietary choices; in medicine, randomized control trials are the gold standard for determining whether a causal relationship exists between an intervention,[67] but there was only one relevant randomized control trial available at the time. I'll share the details of that trial shortly, but first let's look at another meta-analysis.

In 2017, a different group of researchers constructed a meta-analysis in an attempt to answer the question of whether or not there was a relationship between diet and depression. Twenty-one studies from 2 databases met the criteria to be included in the meta-analysis. These studies consisted of 11 cohort studies, 6 cross-sectional studies, and 4 case-control studies.[68]

The results of the study suggested that diets character-ized by high intakes of fruit, vegetables, whole grain, fish, olive oil, low-fat dairy and antioxidants and low intakes of animal foods were associated with a decreased risk of depression, while diets characterized by high consumption of red and/or processed meat, refined grains, sweets, high-fat dairy products, butter, potatoes and high-fat gravy, and low intakes of fruits and vegetables were associated with an increased risk of depression. At the study's conclusion, the researchers who conducted this meta-analysis expressed the grave need for additional, reputable data, stating that more randomized controlled trials and cohort studies were "urgently" required to confirm their findings. [68]

Now let's look at the details of the only randomized controlled trial cited in these two meta-analyses.

The study took a group of omnivores and randomly assigned them to one of three groups: a control group that continued to eat an omnivorous diet including daily fish, poultry, and other meat; a group that ate fish, but restricted consumption of other types of meat; and a group that avoided fish, poultry, and other meats.

The three groups implemented the dietary changes for a total of two weeks. At the end of the two-week period, participants in the group that continued to eat an omnivorous diet and the group that ate fish but restricted other types of meat did not show significant improvements in mood scores. On the other hand, the group that avoided fish, poultry, and other types of meat reported improvements in mood scores, suggesting that consuming a diet high in meat, fish, and poultry may negatively impact mental state.[69]

If you're like me, then you probably want to know why. What exactly was it about these different diets that led to one group experiencing improvements in mood while the other two groups didn't experience much of a change? Here are two important contributing factors: antioxidants and arachidonic acid. I'll explain.

Antioxidants

Researchers wanted to find out the relative levels of antioxidants in fruits, vegetables, and other plant foods compared to the level of antioxidants in other foods such as dairy, eggs, and meat. They found that plant-based foods contain significantly more antioxidants than non-plant foods. For perspective, foods of plant origin had an average of 11.57 mmol of antioxidants per 100 grams of food while foods of animal origin had an average of 0.18 mmol of antioxidants per 100 grams of food.[70]

Now that we've established that foods of plant origin generally contain more antioxidants than foods of animal origin, let's discuss the role that antioxidants play in mental health.

In order to produce energy, a process called oxidative phosphorylation takes place in the mitochondria of our cells. Free radicals, which are highly unstable and very reactive substances, are produced as a by-product of this process. Free radicals are important for normal physiological functions, such as protecting cells from infections by destroying invading microbes. Under normal circumstances, free radicals, which are sometimes referred to as pro-oxidants, are kept in check by antioxidants.

The pro-oxidant/antioxidant balance is critical to optimal health. When this balance is disturbed by an increase in the production of free radicals or a decrease in antioxidants, free radicals can cause oxidative damage, altering the expression of our genes and negatively impacting the viability of our DNA.[71]

Because the brain uses large amounts of oxygen and generates free radicals as a result, it is extremely vulnerable to oxidative damage. Through a variety of different mechanisms,[72] both increased free radical formation and decreased antioxidant status have been linked with mental health concerns such as anxiety, depression, bipolar disorder, and schizophrenia.[71]

Research demonstrates that increasing antioxidant stores of people with anxiety, depression, bipolar disorder, and schizophrenia led to reduced anxiety and depression levels,[73] reduced depression in bipolar disorder,[72] and an impairment in the course of psychotic symptoms, especially persecutory delusions, respectively.[74]

The fact that research demonstrates that individuals who avoid consumption of fish, poultry, and other types of meat have significantly better antioxidant statuses than otherwise healthy omnivores,[75] and the fact that higher antioxidant status is associated with improved mental health explain, at least partially, why omnivores who avoided fish, poultry, and meat for two weeks in our randomized controlled trial experienced such significant improvements in mental health.

The interesting part about this research is that there is a clear correlation between consumption of antioxidants from food sources and both decreased risk of being diagnosed with and improvements in symptoms pertaining to mental health conditions,[76,77] but the research does not show a consistent correlation between antioxidant intake from dietary supplementation and improvements in mental health.[77] This suggests that, if you want to experience the mental health benefits associated with increased antioxidant intake, it is best to consume those antioxidants in the form of a plant-rich diet.

Arachidonic Acid

Now let's look at arachidonic acid, the second major contributing factor to the fact that omnivores who removed fish, poultry, and other forms of meat from their diets experienced improved mental health.

Arachidonic acid (ARA) is a polyunsaturated omega-6 fatty acid that plays a crucial role in the body's signaling for pain and inflammation.[78] ARA is generally considered to be a pro-inflammatory fatty acid. It is converted in the body into compounds that play important roles in activating the inflammatory response such as prostaglandins.

Our bodies make ARA from linoleic acid, a shorter omega-6 fatty acid found in nuts, seeds, and their oils. We also get pre-formed ARA from our diets when we consume animal products such as fish, chicken, beef, pork, other meat, eggs, cheese, and dairy. Because some inflammation is essential to life, our bodies need some ARA to properly function, but too much can significantly affect both physical and mental health.

What does ARA have to do with mental health? I'll explain, but in order to understand my explanation, you need to understand the basics of omega-3 fatty acids.

There are 11 different types of omega-3 fatty acids, but the three most important omega-3s in human physiology are alpha-linolenic acid (ALA), eicosapentaenoic acid (EPA), and docosahexaenoic acid (DHA). ALA is mostly found in plant-based foods like walnuts and flax seeds and is converted in the body to EPA and DHA; while the conversion rates are not extremely high and are dependent upon factors like genetics, sex, age, and diet, the body does convert ALA to EPA and DHA. Outside of this conversion, EPA and DHA are mostly found in fatty fish and certain species of algae. Omega-3 fatty acids have anti-inflammatory effects on the body.[79]

In explaining the effects of ARA on mental health, we'll be looking specifically at ARA and EPA. A related process to what we will be describing occurs with DHA,[80] but research suggests that it's EPA that is most relevant to mood modulation, not DHA.[81] To simplify this explanation, think about ARA and EPA as two people who each have a toddler, and both toddlers want a specific toy. Both parents want to get the toy for their toddlers because they want the specific end result of seeing the joy and excitement on their faces, so they both go to the store with the intent of purchasing this toy. The two parents arrive at the store at the same time, and they find that there is only one toy remaining. Only one of the parents is able to leave the store with the toy and experience the end result of an overjoyed toddler.

Here's how ARA and EPA are similar to these parents: Since ARA and EPA are similar in size and can bind to many of the same enzymes, when we eat foods that contain pre-formed ARA, the pro-inflammatory ARA competes with anti-inflammatory EPA to bind to certain enzymes.[69] Only one of the two can bind to the enzyme at a time and accomplish their specific end result. When ARA succeeds in binding to the enzyme, the result is an increase in the production of pro-inflammatory metabolites like prostaglandins, leading to an increase in the levels of inflammation in the body.

In addition to leading to an increased risk for inflammation-based chronic diseases, this process leads to increased risk for mood disorders like depression and bipolar disorder. We believe this is because prostaglandins alter the rate of blood flow to the brain and/or lead to a decrease in brain-derived neurotrophic factor, which, as a reminder, is a protein that plays an important role in the survival, growth, maturation, and maintenance of brain and nerve cells.[82,83]

To summarize, we established that pro-inflammatory ARA and anti-inflammatory EPA have opposing effects and that higher levels of ARA can lead to an inflammatory state that increases the risk for and severity of symptoms in mood disorders like depression and bipolar disorder. To keep this risk low, it's important to make sure that your intake of omega-6 fatty acids isn't extremely higher than your intake of omega-3 fatty acids.

In the realm of animal foods, fish and some types of seafood contain high amounts of omega-3 fatty acids in addition to the arachidonic acid that they contain. As a result, omega-3 fatty acids oppose the effects of ARA in the diets of omnivores who eat fish regularly and consume comparatively low amounts of other meat. We believe this is the reason why some research shows that omnivores who eat fish regularly report improved moods compared to omnivores who do not eat fish regularly.[69]

In spite of the mental health benefits that are clearly associated with omega-3 fatty acid consumption, our randomized controlled trial showed that omnivores who temporarily restricted fish, poultry, and other meat experienced dramatically improved mood scores compared to omnivores who ate fish but restricted other meat and those who did not restrict any types of meat from their diets. Why was that?

Well, there are a few possible explanations. One such reason is the bioaccumulation of heavy metals and toxic chemicals as we go up the food chain. In other words, plants and small organisms like plankton take up these metals and chemicals, and then small fish eat these small organisms. As these small fish eat more and more of these organisms, more heavy metals and chemicals accumulate in their bodies. Medium-sized fish then eat these small fish, even larger fish eat those fish, and the levels of heavy metals and chemicals in the bodies of the fish are compounded as we move higher and higher up the food chain. When humans consume fish, the accumulated metals and chemicals are then introduced into our bodies.

Researchers wanted to evaluate the effects of heavy metals on the health of people consuming seafood. Study participants did not have any positive risk factors for cardiovascular disease and their fish and other seafood consumption levels were under the World Health Organization's (WHO) provisional tolerable weekly intake, a value set by the WHO which is viewed as the acceptable level of a toxic metal that can be consumed on a weekly basis without the person consuming it experiencing adverse health effects.

At the end of their study, researchers found that eating even a moderate amount of seafood could result in negative effects on the body such as atherosclerosis and negative changes in the lipid profile. Researchers concluded that these negative effects were likely attributable to the participants' arsenic and mercury exposure from the seafood, indicating that we may have overestimated the amount of heavy metals that humans can safely consume.[84]

This research is relevant to mental health because chronic heavy metal exposure has been found to play important roles in many mental health conditions. Regarding these two metals in particular, evidence suggests that exposure to both arsenic and mercury is linked to depression[85,86] and suicide risk.[86,87] Additionally, arsenic exposure has been linked to behavioral changes,[85] and mercury exposure has been linked to anxiety.[86]

In essence, the improvements seen in the mood scores of those who avoided fish, poultry, and other meat could have been due to the fact that the arachidonic acid and heavy metal content of fish in the group that consumed fish but avoided other types of meat counteracted the beneficial effects of the omega-3 fatty acids in the fish.

This explains a lot, but, considering the fact that omega-3 fatty acids have been associated in quite a few studies with mood improvements, it still doesn't explain why the group in our randomized controlled trial that avoided fish, poultry, and other meat experienced mood improvements above the other groups, especially when their total omega-3 fatty acid consumption was so low.

Research does demonstrate that individuals who do not consume any fish or other meat at all have low baseline levels of omega-3 fatty acids, similar to omnivores who don't eat much fish,[88] but their mood scores are much better than omnivores. This is because, when it comes to omega-6 and omega-3 fatty acids, the ratio of omega-3s to omega-6s is more important than the actual amount of each fatty acid type. While the ideal omega-6 to omega-3 ratio is 4 to 1 or lower, some estimates report that the ratio in the standard American diet may be anywhere from 15:1 to 16.7:1.[89]

During our randomized controlled trial, ARA levels fell to 0.00 grams after 2 weeks in the group that avoided all meat. People who habitually restrict the consumption of dairy, eggs, and meat including poultry and fish have very low to non-existent levels of ARA. Although our bodies do synthesize ARA from linoleic acid when we eat nuts, seeds, and their oils, very little linoleic acid is actually converted into ARA; furthermore, some research suggests that eating a diet that is higher in linoleic acid leads to a down-regulation of the ARA pathway, which results in reduced conversion of linoleic acid to ARA.[69,90]

Therefore, because people eating minimal processed foods and restricting dietary intake of fish, poultry, and other meat have extremely low ARA levels, they need less dietary omega-3 to balance their omega-6s than an omnivore would. In other words, low baseline omega-3 fatty acid levels may not be as much of a problem in these people as it is in omnivores.

We saw that the body makes EPA and DHA from ALA. The process of synthesizing EPA and DHA from this omega-3 fatty acid is limited, however, to 8-20% for conversion of ALA to EPA and 1-9% for the conversion of ALA to DHA. Researchers noted that in spite of their very low or virtually absent dietary intake of EPA and DHA, those who avoid dietary consumption of fish, poultry, and other meat do not exhibit clinical signs of deficiency.[91] They further stated that, although we do not currently understand all of the details surrounding omega-3 needs for individuals who do not eat meat, their recommendation is that these people prophylactically reduce their intake of omega-6 fatty acids and consume double the current adequate intake of ALA if they aren't consuming any direct sources if EPA and DHA.

For perspective, the adequate intake of ALA is currently set at 2 grams per day. Doubling this value would mean consuming the equivalent of 2 tablespoons of ground flaxseeds per day, as each tablespoon of flax seed contains 2 grams of ALA.[92] For those who have increased needs (pregnant or breastfeeding women) or impaired conversion ability (older people and those with diabetes or another chronic disease), researchers recommended a plant-based (algae) omega-3 supplement containing 200-300 mg per day of EPA and DHA. This research showed that those on the plant-based diet who made these changes responded well to these relatively low doses of supplemental omega-3s and were able to benefit from the omega-3s in the algae oil[91] while avoiding increased cardiovascular and other health risks due to heavy metals like arsenic and mercury in fish, and increased neurological, immunological, and repro-ductive risk in offspring associated with increased body burden from chemicals such as polychlorinated biphenyls and other endocrine-disrupting compounds frequently found in fish.[93,94]

Long-term Effects of Such a Diet

Now that we've thoroughly analyzed the beneficial mental health effects that the individuals who completely restricted meat for a two-week period experienced in our randomized controlled trial, we need to evaluate whether or not this type of diet results in improved mental health in the long run.

Since the publication of the 2-week randomized controlled trial, researchers have conducted longer relevant randomized controlled trials. In 2010, researchers conducted a randomized controlled trial where they took a group of 113 people working for a particular company and randomized them into two different groups.[95] They provided the intervention group with instructions regarding preparing meals without the use of dairy, eggs, fish, poultry, and other meat (plant-based) and the control group received no instruction. The company's cafeteria also offered plant-based options such as lentil soup, minestrone soup, veggie burgers, portabella mushroom sandwiches, salads, bean burritos, and rice and beans, and all participants were asked to take a multivitamin in order to meet their requirements for vitamin B12. Researchers followed the participants for a total of 22 weeks.

At the end of the study, participants eating the plant-based diet reported a significant increase in their overall satisfaction with their diet compared to the control group, a significant decrease in the cost of food purchases, better sleep than usual, and, most relevant to our current discussion, the plant-based group reported a significant improvement in their mental health over the course of the 22 weeks, whereas the control group did not report an improvement in their mental health.

Researchers conducted another related randomized controlled trial in 2015.[96] This time the study was conducted at 10 corporate sites with 292 participants over the course of 18 weeks. Again, participants were randomized into an intervention group that received plant-based instruction and a control group that did not receive any instruction, and participants at the intervention sites were asked to take a multivitamin. At the end of the 18 weeks, participants who ate a plant-based diet reported significant improvements in depression, anxiety, fatigue, emotional wellbeing, and daily functioning because of emotional health compared with the group that received no dietary instruction.

These two longer randomized controlled trials demonstrated that consuming a plant-based diet resulted in significant improvements in mental health and energy levels, and they also demonstrated that such a diet, when intelligently implemented, could be both enjoyable and cost-effective. The longer of these studies, however, only spanned the course of about five and a half months, so neither study provided enough information to draw conclusions regarding potential negative effects associated with being on this type of diet for years.

To evaluate the long-term effects of restricting fish, poultry, and other meat from the diet, researchers assessed a group of adult Seventh-day Adventists, a Christian group that is known for its emphasis on health and whose parishioners make up the only Blue Zone® (region of the world where people live much longer than average) in America.[97] Approximately one-third of Seventh-day Adventists eat no meat, making them the ideal group in which to study the long-term effects of such a diet on mental health and other chronic diseases. In a cross-sectional study assessing the health of Adventist participants, researchers demonstrated that individuals who habitually avoided meat reported significantly less depression, anxiety, stress, and negative emotions than omnivores.

To return to our discussion on omega-3 fatty acids, this study was interesting because its results actually suggested that improved mood was associated with lower levels of EPA, DHA, and ARA, and higher levels of ALA and linoleic acid.[98]

This study isn't the only one to suggest that improved mood is associated with lower levels of the omega-3 fatty acids EPA and DHA. A 10-year, prospective cohort study that looked at 54,632 women who were between the ages of 50 and 77 and showed no signs of depression at the beginning of the 10 years found that long-chain omega-3 fatty acids from fish do not protect against depression; in this study, higher ALA and linoleic acid intake were instead found to reduce depression risk.[99]

Other research supports this idea as well. In a clinical trial that lasted one year, obese participants were randomly assigned to either a low-carbohydrate (animal-based) diet or a low-fat (plant-based) diet. At the end of the year, both groups lost similar amounts of weight, but the low-fat group reported dramatic decreases in depression, feelings of dejection, anxiety, anger, hostility, stress, mental confusion, mood disturbance, and fatigue. They also reported increases in vigor and energy compared to the low-carbohydrate group.[100]

These results are consistent with research that has demonstrated that while high-carbohydrate intake can increase serotonin synthesis, fat and protein intake reduce serotonin concentrations in the brain, negatively impacting mood.[101]

I'll explain the mechanism of action for you. Because tryptophan is the amino acid that is converted into serotonin in the body, the rate at which the brain produces serotonin depends largely upon the levels of tryptophan in the blood. Tryptophan uses the same means of transportation from the blood into the brain as other amino acids, and this results in tryptophan needing to compete with more prevalent amino acids, such as tyrosine, methionine, phenylalanine, isoleucine, leucine, and valine for transport into the brain.[102]

The types of foods that we eat directly affect blood concentrations of tryptophan and indirectly affect serotonin production and release. When we consume carbohy-drate-rich foods, the body secretes insulin, which results in the amino acids isoleucine, leucine, and valine (collectively referred to as branched-chain amino acids or BCAAs) being taken up out of the circulation into the muscles. Because the BCAAs are comparatively abundant in protein, com-prising 15-20% of the proteins that we consume,[103] this reduction in the BCAAs by means of insulin results in an increased ratio of plasma tryptophan to plasma concentra-tions of the other amino acids and an increased likelihood that tryptophan will actually be transported into the brain for serotonin synthesis.

In contrast, when you consume a diet that is pro-tein-heavy and restricts carbohydrate consumption, we see a lower ratio of tryptophan to the other amino acids in the plasma,[102] which results in lower levels of trypto-phan being available to be transported into the brain for serotonin synthesis.[104]

To summarize, high-carbohydrate intake results in insu-lin secretion, which decreases BCAA concentrations in the plasma, and increases the ratio of tryptophan to other amino acids. This increases the likelihood of tryptophan binding to the appropriate protein and being carried into the brain for serotonin synthesis. Consuming foods that are high in fat and protein and low in carbohydrates does not have the same effect on BCAAs, resulting in a lower ratio of tryptophan to the other amino acids, less tryptophan being carried into the brain, reduced serotonin synthesis and release, and an increase in symptoms associated with low serotonin such as increased cravings and depressed mood.[103,104]

Plant-Based Diets

Through analyzing the research and drawing conclusions based on my clinical experiences, I've found that certain foods are correlated to improved mental (and overall) well-being, while others tend to be associated with increased risk for mental health disorders. I've discussed animal-based foods and arachidonic acid at great length because the basis of the P7 Protocol™ Diet is a plant-based diet and, when it comes to addressing diet in the context of mental health, animal-based foods like dairy, eggs, and meat tend to be surrounded by the most controversy; no one really argues when I say that eating your vegetables results in improved mental and overall health. Before we talk about the foods included in the P7 Protocol™ Diet, I'd like to address a few myths concerning plant-based diets in general.

Debunking Myths

One of the main claims against any diet that restricts the consumption of animal-based foods is that it leads to macro- and micronutrient deficiencies. This is partially because early studies on plant-based diets were conducted on individuals who consumed very restricted diets; in other words, they were eating this way because they couldn't afford to eat anything else and their diets consisted of only a few different foods. In developed countries today, however, plant-based diets consist of far greater variety, making it far more difficult to actually become nutrient-deficient while on a well-planned plant-based diet. Nevertheless, there are a few key nutrients that are frequently cited when it comes to plant-based diets, some of which are legitimate concerns. I'll share the most frequently cited nutrients over the next several sections.

Protein

The macronutrient that is most frequently cited is—you probably guessed it—protein. The belief that plant-based diets are deficient in protein is founded upon the misconceptions that plants do not contain much protein and that human beings need exorbitant amounts of protein to survive.

The United States Department of Agriculture recommends that individuals above the age of 19 consume at least 0.8 grams of protein per kilogram of body weight per day. According to these guidelines, a person who weighs 125 pounds should consume at least 45 grams of protein per day, while a person who weighs 165 pounds should consume at least 60 grams of protein per day. For perspective, one cup of cooked lentils contains about 18 grams of protein and one cup of cooked kidney beans contains about 15 grams of protein. It's easy to think about legumes, nuts, and seeds as containing protein, but what about plant-based foods that we don't typically think about as being high in protein? Well, one large baked potato and a cup of cooked green peas contain about 16 grams of protein. That's almost half the recommended daily protein intake for a 125-pound person and almost one-third of the recommended daily protein intake for a 165-pound person.

In human physiology, there appears to be a difference between plant-based proteins and animal-based proteins. Research demonstrates that diets high in animal protein increase cancer death risk and overall mortality tremendously by increasing something called insulin-like growth factor 1, whereas plant-based protein didn't have that effect.[105] In addition to supporting the fact that plant-based proteins promote increased longevity compared to animal-based protein, research also supports the fact that plant-based foods contain adequate amounts of protein. A cross-sectional study looking at 71,751 people who participated in the Adventist Health Study showed that adherents to a plant-based diet consistently met and exceeded their daily protein recommendations. In this large study, participants on a plant-based diet consumed, on average, 70.7 grams of protein per day, while those who adhered to an omnivorous diet averaged 74.7 grams of protein per day,[106] demonstrating that humans are fully capable of meeting and even exceeding their protein needs without consuming meat.

Legumes

Legumes are plants or the fruit or seed of plants in the Leguminosae or Fabaceae family. To keep it simple, think of legumes as beans, peas, lentils, and peanuts. There are a few popular diets that limit or completely prohibit the consumption of legumes. The reason that is frequently cited is the fact that they contain "anti-nutrients" like lectins, enzyme inhibitors, and phytic acid. If you're familiar with or you've ever adhered to one of these diets, then given the fact that legumes absolutely do contain anti-nutrients, you're probably wondering whether or not we should consume legumes. Before you make a decision, I'll explain the backstory.

First of all, anti-nutrients are natural or synthetic compounds that are found in a variety of foods. They limit or inhibit absorption of valuable nutrients including vitamins and minerals. Lectins, also known as phytohemagglutinins, are proteins that bind carbohydrates and that are present in most plants, including seeds, grains, and legumes. They are also found to varying degrees in tomatoes, potatoes, string beans, carrots, apples, grapefruit, cantaloupe, raspberries, blackberries, garlic, marjoram, mushrooms, coffee beans, and other foods.[107]

The alarm concerning lectins is mainly due to a case study recorded in the British Medical journal in 1999. The case study alleged that in 1988, a hospital served kidney beans to a group of people and they ended up vomiting and with additional symptoms of food poisoning. When they could not isolate any bacteria or other pathogen that may have caused the gastroenteritis, they began to assess the kidney beans and found them to contain large amounts of lectins. This led to additional research on lectins and a variety of people and movements extrapolating the results of this hospital experience to say that we should completely avoid legumes.[108]

Looking at the latest research, it is clear that lectins can be harmful in large amounts. However, it turned out that the kidney beans that were served at the hospital in 1988 contained abnormally high amounts of lectins because they were undone. Research shows that lectins in foods are mostly deactivated or destroyed by cooking. In fact, one study showed that boiling soybeans in water for as little as 5-10 minutes virtually eliminated all lectin activity.[109-111] Therefore, as long as we are cooking our beans before eating them, the concern regarding dietary lectins from legumes is a non-issue.

Let's briefly look beyond lectins to other types of anti-nutrients. Anti-nutrients that fall under the class of enzyme inhibitors, such as are commonly found in legumes, can prevent enzymes from breaking down fats and protein in the way they normally would. Enzyme inhibitors are made significantly less active by cooking, boiling, or sprouting,[112] and chronic ingestion of residual levels is unlikely to pose risks to human health.[113]

Similarly, phytic acid or phytate, found in both legumes and grains, has been shown to inhibit the body's ability to absorb minerals. Phytic acid also has potent antioxidant properties and has been shown to lower the incidence of colon cancer and protect against inflammatory bowel disease.[114] Phytic acid, like lectins and enzyme inhibitors, are made significantly less active by cooking, boiling, sprouting, or leavening such as in baking leavened bread.[112,115] Furthermore, gut bacteria such as *Lactobacillus rhamnosus* and *Lactobacillus plantarum* have been shown to produce the enzyme phytase resulting in the degradation of phytates.[116]

To reduce the amount of anti-nutrients consumed, I recommend that my patients soak their dried legumes overnight and discard the water before cooking. This also improves the digestibility of legumes and tends to reduce the incidence of bloating and flatulence that some people experience when eating beans. I also recommend sprouting legumes whenever possible; avoiding the consumption of raw grains, such as raw oatmeal in smoothies; and limiting the consumption of unleavened bread, because grains, like legumes, need to be cooked or leavened in order to deactivate the anti-nutrients that are present in them.

Carbohydrates

Another claim that is frequently brought against plant-based diets is that the consumption of large amounts of carbohydrates is associated with insulin spikes and erratic blood sugar levels.

Contrary to this alarmingly common belief, several studies have actually demonstrated that people avoiding meat have lower incidences of insulin resistance than their omnivorous counterparts and that the degree of insulin sensitivity appears to be correlated with the amount of years for which they've consumed such a diet; in other words, those who do not eat meat tend to have lower levels of insulin resistance than those who do and the bodies of those who avoid meat become more and more sensitive to insulin as time goes on for as long as they adhere to this diet.[117-119]

Furthermore, a 20-year-long study conducted on 40,475 non-diabetic individuals demonstrated that those on a low-carbohydrate diet that was high in animal-based proteins and fats were twice as likely to develop type 2 diabetes than those on a low-carbohydrate diet that was high in plant-based proteins and fats. This study indicated that, as far as dietary risk factors are concerned, our risk of insulin resistance and type two diabetes may have slightly less to do with carbohydrates than we originally thought and may be more closely associated with the source of our proteins and fats, with animal-based sources leading to an increased risk and plant-based sources either showing no association at all, or as in the case of men under the age of 65, being associated with a decreased risk of insulin resistance and type 2 diabetes.[120]

Iron and Zinc

Two potential micronutrient deficiencies that are frequently cited are iron are zinc. Because the plant-based diet features increased intake of phytate-containing legumes and grains and reduced intake of meat compared to the standard American diet, some researchers have expressed concerns about the absorption of iron and zinc while on a plant-based diet.

Regarding iron, research shows that while people who avoid meat often have lower ferritin levels than omnivores despite the fact that the total iron intake between the two groups is comparable, the differences between hemoglobin levels in the two groups are small and are rarely associated with anemia.[121]

High-quality data on objectively observable zinc deficiency as marked by low serum zinc concentrations in people avoiding meat is limited, but the data we do have suggest no difference in zinc concentrations of children and adults avoiding meat and omnivores. There is some evidence that adolescents who avoid meat may have lower zinc concentrations than adolescent omnivores.[121]

Research regarding zinc concentrations in individuals avoiding meat is particularly conflicting because many studies look at data from individuals living in or who have recently migrated from underdeveloped nations, and these people may be predisposed to iron and zinc deficiency because of non-dietary factors such as chronic inflammation, parasitic infections, overweight, and genetic hemoglobin disorders.[121]

The current recommended daily allowance (RDA) for iron is 8mg per day for men and 18 mg per day for women ages 19-50 (8 mg per day for women ages 51 and older). The RDA for zinc is 8 mg for women and 11 mg for men. The Adventist Health Study demonstrated that omnivores averaged 20 mg of iron and 11.9 mg of zinc per day while adherents to a plant-based diet averaged 22.2 mg of iron and 11.3 mg of zinc per day.[106]

To summarize, although individuals who avoid meat have been demonstrated to have lower ferritin, adverse health effects of lower iron and zinc absorption have not been demonstrated with varied, plant-based diets consumed in developed countries.[122] If you are concerned about iron or zinc deficiency, limiting the consumption of anti-nutrients by cooking or sprouting legumes and boiling, cooking, sprouting, or leavening grains, avoiding the consumption of tannin-rich teas and coffee, consuming vitamin-C rich foods with meals to enhance iron absorption, and consuming foods that are fortified can all reduce the risk of deficiency and the need for supplementation.

Calcium

Calcium is another potential micronutrient deficiency that is frequently referenced. Calcium is of concern because low levels can increase the risk of osteoporosis and fractures. If you assume for a moment that adherents to a plant-based diet actually do consume low amounts of calcium, you would likely conclude that they must have low bone mineral density as a result and they must be at increased risk for osteoporosis. On the contrary, however, research demonstrates that those who eat a balanced, plant-based diet do not have an increased risk of fracture or osteoporosis.[123]

Evidence suggests that adherents to high-fat diets such as the Ketogenic diet are at increased risk for osteoporosis and fractures. This is likely due to the highly acidic nature of the diet. Researchers believe that plant-based adherents do not exhibit increased risk of osteoporosis because of their diets' low acid load. Low acid load is correlated with lower bone resorption, higher bone mineral density, and higher intake of potassium-rich foods such as fruits and vegetables. Studies show that the acid load in plant-based diets is either minimal or completely absent, while the omnivorous standard American diet tends to produce 50 to 70 mEq of acid per day. The low acid content of plant-based diets protects those who eat them from osteoporosis and fractures.[123]

Vitamin D

Vitamin D is another potential micronutrient deficiency that is frequently cited when discussing plant-based diets. Like calcium, vitamin D is important for bone health and osteoporosis prevention, but vitamin D is also important for mental health. Sub-optimal vitamin D levels are associated with minor and major depression,[124] and research demonstrates that preventing vitamin D deficiency in early childhood may reduce the incidence of schizophrenia.[125]

Natural dietary sources of vitamin D are mainly limited to fish liver oils, fatty fish, and egg yolks, and additional dietary sources include fortified milks and cereals.

Aside from dietary sources of vitamin D, our bodies convert cholesterol into vitamin D when we expose large portions of our bare skin to ultraviolet-B (UV-B) light. Factors that affect sunlight needs in order to make vitamin D include skin color, with individuals who have darker skin needing more sunlight exposure compared to individuals with fairer skin; time of day, with exposure at midday resulting in greater production of vitamin D in a given time period compared to exposure at sunrise or sunset; amount of skin exposed, with larger portions of bare skin exposed resulting in greater vitamin D production; season, with summer resulting in greater vitamin D production and winter resulting in less vitamin D production; and distance from the equator, with individuals living closer to the equator producing more vitamin D on average compared to individuals living farther from the equator.

Because sunscreen blocks UV-B rays, its use impairs the body's ability to produce vitamin D. Most sunscreens also contain neurotoxic and endocrine-disrupting chemicals, many of which have been linked to disruption of reproductive hormone function, thyroid gland function, and behavioral changes.[126-127] For example, preclinical research suggests that octyl methoxycinnamate, also known as octinoxate, can negatively impact thyroid function at multiple levels of the HPT axis and can inhibit the release of neurotransmitters in the brain.[127] To limit exposure to these toxic chemicals, I typically recommend that if patients absolutely must use sunscreen, that they use mineral-based sunscreens such as zinc oxide- and titanium dioxide-based sunscreens. These sunscreens still block UVB rays, but their ingredients tend to be less toxic.

Let's return to our discussion of vitamin D. The blood test that we typically use to evaluate vitamin D levels tests for 25-hydroxycholecalciferol, also known as 25-hydroxyvitamin D. The Endocrine Society defines vitamin D insufficiency as a 25hydroxyvitamin D level between 21 and

29 ng/mL and vitamin D deficiency as a 25hydroxyvitamin D blood level below 20 ng/mL.[128] Research demonstrates that 77% of Americans have vitamin D levels below 30 ng/mL, indicating that only 23% of Americans have vitamin D levels within the normal range.[129]

Because of the widespread prevalence of vitamin D deficiency among both individuals on an animal-based and a plant-based diet, I typically recommend that my patients supplement with vitamin D in order to achieve and maintain adequate levels, regardless of the type of diet they consume.

Vitamin B12

Perhaps the most frequently cited micronutrient when it comes to objections to consuming a plant-based diet is vitamin B12. Everyone seems to have an opinion and it can be difficult to know what is true. Over the next several paragraphs, we'll get to the bottom of the B12 quandary.

First of all, neither plants nor animals make B12; it's actually made by bacteria. Animals consume bacteria, humans eat the meat of these animals, and that's how omnivores get their B12. Although B12 is a water-soluble vitamin, we're able to store it in the liver for long periods of time. In fact, if you were to stop consuming all sources of B12 today, you would still have enough stored up to last you 3-5 years.[130] Vitamin B12 is extremely important to health because deficiencies can lead to elevations in an amino acid called homocysteine, which negatively affects mental health and causes increased levels of inflammation, neurological concerns, and cardiovascular risk. As we've previously discussed, this is because the body uses vitamins B6, B9, and B12 to convert homocysteine back into another amino acid called methionine. Under normal circumstances, methionine then becomes S-adenosylmethionine, which is important for neurotransmitter function, DNA synthesis, and a host of other processes.

The 71,751-person Adventist Health Study demonstrated that 95% of participants who avoided meat consumption had similar B12 levels to omnivores, which is likely a result of B12 production by gut bacteria and consumption of B12-fortified foods such as cereals, nut milk, soymilk, and nutritional yeast. The bottom 5th percentile of participants who were studied, however, had very low B12 levels.[106] Low B12 levels are typically due to low dietary intake of meat, B12-fortified foods, or B12 supplements; insufficient gastric acid levels due to old age or acid-blocking medication; and/or poor B12 production by gut bacteria.

Knowing all of the health benefits associated with being on a plant-based diet as well as the fact that those who have eaten this way for longer periods of time without consuming B12-fortified foods or supplementing with B12 do have lower levels of this vitamin, researchers set out to find the optimal levels and method of supplementation in people on this diet. What they found was that dietary B12 is separated from the proteins that we eat by digestive enzymes in the stomach where it binds to a carrier protein called transcobalamin I (TCN1). TCN1 is secreted in the saliva and enters the stomach after chewing and swallowing. As the partially-digested food enters the small intestine, B12 is released from TCN1 and binds to intrinsic factor (which is initially produced by the parietal cells in the stomach) where it is carried to the last part of the small intestine, the ileum, and absorbed into the bloodstream.[131]

We know that the body can only absorb about 1.5–2 µg of dietary B12 per meal before the transporters become saturated. There is, however, a certain amount of B12, about 1% of total B12 when higher doses are consumed, that is absorbed through passive diffusion across the gastrointestinal mucosa. This means that taking a large dose of 1 mg results in the absorption of approximately 11.5-12 µg, about 5 times the United States Institute of Medicine's RDA and about 3 times the European Food Safety Authority's more conservative adequate intake (AI) requirement guidelines of 4 µg per day.[131]

Assuming that the absorption rate of approximately 1% is maintained at even higher dosages than 1 mg and keeping in mind the body's ability to store absorbed B12, some physicians have recommended that those who want to enjoy the health benefits of a plant-based diet without allowing their B12 levels to fall to suboptimal values take at least 2500 µg (2.5 mg) of B12 sublingually once per week, which averages out to approximately 4 µg of B12 per day.

As long as they supplement with a form of vitamin B12 that is appropriate for their genetics, I have no preference regarding the manner in which my patients supplement with vitamin B12; they can do so by taking a mega-dose once weekly or they can do so by supplementing twice daily. If my patients choose to take a high-quality multivitamin that contains vitamin B12 on a daily basis, I specifically recommend that they take their multivitamin in divided doses with two separate meals several hours apart since this maximizes absorption and makes it more likely that they will meet their daily requirements.

My Professional Opinion of Plant-Based Diets

My professional opinion of plant-based diets that consist of whole, minimally processed foods aligns with the official position of the Academy of Nutrition and Dietetics. They expressed the conclusion of my research well when they stated that "appropriately planned vegetarian, including vegan, diets are healthful, nutritionally adequate, and may provide health benefits for the prevention and treatment of certain diseases. These diets are appropriate for all stages of the life cycle, including pregnancy, lactation, infancy, childhood, adolescence, older adulthood, and for athletes."[132]

The Academy of Nutrition and Dietetics continued on to report that "low intake of saturated fat and high intakes of vegetables, fruits, whole grains, legumes, soy products, nuts, and seeds (all rich in fiber and phytochemicals) are characteristics of vegetarian and vegan diets that produce lower total and low-density lipoprotein cholesterol levels and better serum glucose control. These factors contribute to reduction of chronic disease."[132]

The P7 Protocol™ Diet

Now that we're clear on the facts concerning the main objections to plant-based diets in general, I'll discuss the specifics of the P7 Protocol™ Diet.

I've seen both in the literature and in my own clinical experience that the components of the P7 Protocol™ Diet, a diet that is individualized, varied, plant-based, and focuses on whole-foods, are an incredibly important therapeutic tool for people experiencing mental health concerns. This is because it helps restore balance to the gastrointestinal tract and microbiome, is rich in antioxidants and phytochemicals, supports optimal neurotransmitter production and function and a healthy fatty acid profile, minimizes neuroinflammation, and supports optimal hormone levels, liver function, and detoxification.

Individualized

Firstly, the P7 Protocol™ Diet is individualized. In other words, it allows room for both personal preferences and individual differences. I ensure that each diet is individualized by starting each patient off with my Elimination and Challenge Protocol. This allows us to identify otherwise healthy foods (like oranges) to which they may be reacting because of poor gastrointestinal health. By eliminating and then reintroducing foods into the diet in order to test them, we are able to construct a dietary plan that is individualized to each patient's needs.

The diet is also individualized in that I make specific nutrient recommendations based on the physical and overall health of each patient. For example, I may make recommendations to limit iodine intake and balance it with selenium if my patient has Hashimoto's thyroiditis, or to limit consumption of foods in the Brassica family like cabbage and Brussels sprouts if my patient has hypothyroidism without the autoimmune component, or some other recommendation that is unique to the specific patient because of his or her current state of health.

Varied

If you have never eaten this way, you may be tempted to think that such a diet is mundane and lacks variety. When I recommend this diet to patients, I get the whole spectrum of reactions, from "So will I only be eating salad?" to "I used to eat that way before and, now that I think about it, I remember feeling great!" and everything in between. The response I get tends to correlate directly with the extent of the person's previous exposure to a plant-based diet.

As demonstrated in the randomized controlled trial I referenced previously where participants reported a significant increase in their overall satisfaction with their diet after restricting their consumption of dairy, eggs, and meat for a total of 22 weeks,[95] when people are properly educated regarding plant-based food preparation, eating this way can be extremely enjoyable as well as health-promoting. Education regarding food preparation is a crucial part of ensuring success when transitioning to a P7 Protocol-compliant lifestyle, because evidence suggests that eating meals that were cooked at home is associated with better diet quality and lower food cost compared to frequently eating out at restaurants,[133] and if you aren't used to preparing foods in this way, you'll likely run out of ideas and either revert back to eating the way you did before or resort to eating out at restaurants.

In addition to being both health-promoting and enjoyable, the P7 Protocol™ Diet is also varied when done correctly. Individuals are not limited to 4 or 5 of the same meals; the possibilities are endless for food combinations. I specifically encourage my patients to eat a variety of different fruits and vegetables in order to ensure adequate and varied nutrient intake, and one way that I help them do that is by encouraging them to make sure that their meals contain foods that are a variety of different colors.

Whole Foods

Not all plant-based diets focus on whole foods. It's completely possible to restrict the consumption of dairy, eggs, and meat and still eat a lot of unhealthy, processed foods. The P7 Protocol™ Diet encourages the consumption of minimally processed, whole foods including fruits, vegetables, nuts, grains, seeds, and legumes and limits the consumption of highly refined and processed foods.

As a general rule for mental health, the less processed a food is, the better. For example, research demonstrates that intake of raw fruits and vegetables significantly predicted higher mental health outcomes when assessing depressive symptoms, anxiety, negative and positive mood, life satisfaction, and flourishing (e.g. living a purposeful life), whereas consumption of processed fruits and vegetables had no association with mental health outcomes.[134]

While heavily processed foods tend to be low in fiber and nutrients, research shows that diets that emphasize whole foods are rich in both fiber and nutrients, and are associated with increases in the diversity of the gastrointestinal microbiome and improvements in gut health. This is important for mental health because dysbiotic flora is associated with elevated levels of pro-inflammatory cytokines, increased oxidative stress, altered gastrointestinal function, and lowered micronutrient and omega-3 fatty acid status,[135] all of which increase the risk of being diagnosed with a variety of mental health disorders, as well as increased symptom severity in the event of diagnosis.

Plant-Based

In addition to the effects of consuming pre-formed arachidonic acid on the omega-6 to omega-3 ratio, which we discussed at length, consumption of dairy, eggs, and meat also results in changes to the microbiome, which can be problematic for mental health.

Researchers took a group of people and gave them two different diets over a given period of time. Participants consumed a diet consisting of meats, eggs, and cheeses for five consecutive days followed by a washout period and then they consumed a diet consisting of grains, legumes, fruits, and vegetables for 5 consecutive days followed by a washout period. Researchers found that the differences in diet over each five-day period led to significant changes in the microbiome. Consumption of the animal-based diet led to a decrease in overall gut microbial diversity and an increase in bile-tolerant microorganisms, including *Biloph-ila wadsworthia*, a bacteria whose presence is known to be capable of triggering inflammatory bowel disease. While minimal changes were noted on the plant-based diet, the rapid changes that were noted while participants were on the animal-based diet, mainly the decrease in microbial diversity and the significant increase in bilophilic microorganisms known to produce gastrointestinal inflammation, are both changes that we know can negatively and significantly impact mental health.[136]

Long-term studies support the therapeutic use of plant-based diets in improving mental health. The P7 Protocol™ Diet can be categorized as a plant-based diet, yet it is not simply plant-based, because the term "plant-based" only suggests that a given diet excludes the consumption of foods from animal sources, such as milk, yogurt, cheese, and other dairy; eggs; and fish, poultry, and other meat.

This diet is more than simply plant-based, as it also excludes the consumption of some substances that are of plant origin, but have been shown to have devastating or otherwise negative effects on mental and overall health, such as alcohol, which promotes the growth of gram-negative bacteria in the gut resulting in endotoxin accumulation, disruption of gastrointestinal barrier function, and increased intestinal permeability,[137] all of which can result in increased hyper-permeability of the gastrointestinal tract to bacterial products[138] and negatively impact the HPA axis and overall mental health; tobacco, which has been identified as a causal risk factor in schizophrenia[139] and is associated with increased risk and earlier onset of psychosis,[140] increased suicidality in bipolar disorder,[141] and increased risk for depression;[142] and other drugs.

Another plant-based substance that has been negatively associated with mental health and should be avoided is caffeine, which is known to induce chemical dependence and is capable of inducing anxiety, mania, and psychosis.[143] Caffeine use can be especially detrimental in patients with panic disorder, performance or social anxiety, bipolar disorder, and schizophrenia.[143-144] Although some observational studies suggest that caffeine intake is associated with improvements in depression and suicide risk,[145-146] a systematic review on the topic suggests that the evidence we now have is insufficient to draw a sound conclusion regarding the relationship between caffeine and depression and suicidality.[143] Furthermore, caffeine is metabolized in the liver by the CYP1A2 enzyme and can therefore interact with other drugs that are metabolized at this enzyme such as medication used to address depression, anxiety, psychosis, mania, and insomnia, leading to an increase in drug-related side effects and complications in medical treatment.[147]

In spite of the observed negative effects of these psychoactive substances on mental health, one could make the case that individuals who use these substances are attempting to self-medicate in order to address their mental health concerns. If this is your argument, then you likely believe that removing these substances would result in a worsening of symptoms. However, in my clinical experience, I've seen the opposite to be true. Psychoactive substances actually complicate the treatment process and make it more difficult to reach treatment goals.

Additionally, research shows that removal of psychoactive substances does not result in a worsening of mental health.[148] In fact, because discontinuing the use of substances can lead to substantial improvements in mental wellbeing and physical health, psychiatrists and other practitioners are actually urged to provide patients with support to discontinue their use.[149]

Whenever indicated, I assist my patients by providing nutritional support and connecting them with therapists as needed in order to facilitate easier transitions throughout the process of discontinuing their use of these psychoactive substances.

Supplements In The P7 Protocol™ Diet

As a part of implementing a successful P7 Protocol™ Diet, I believe that it is important to check markers of vitamin B12 status, vitamin D status, and omega-3 status and supplement in cases of deficiency in order to ensure optimal levels. I actually make these recommendations for many of my patients, regardless of their diet, because

I know that having ample amounts of these nutrients on board can do wonders for the body and that many people, even those not on the P7 Protocol™ Diet, are deficient in one or more of these important nutrients.

In my practice, I also recommend additional indicated, high-quality nutritional supplements to address other components of my patients' health.

Why Are Other Diets Successful?

In light all that I've shared, you should be asking, "If the P7 Protocol™ Diet is truly the ideal diet for addressing my health concerns, then why does research also show that other diets are effective in addressing mental health? Why do study participants on the other diets also get well?"

Here's the hard truth: Research shows that the vast majority of Americans are not consistently meeting the minimum recommendations for nutrient-dense food groups. As examples, over 90% of women between the ages of 19 and 30 had usual intakes below the recommendations for 8 food groups including total fruits, whole fruits, several vegetable subgroups, and whole grains, and over 90% of people in at least half of the age groups who participated in the study were deficient in vegetables. If you are eating the standard American diet (which means you're likely not getting the nutrients you need from the foods you eat) and then I take you off of that diet and put you on a diet that includes far more fruits and vegetables than you were previously eating, don't you think you would see an improvement in your health, regardless of the other components of your diet? You absolutely would.[150]

If you've experienced benefits from adhering to a different diet, it's likely because that diet is more nutrient-dense than the diet you ate previously and making the change helped you to meet or even exceed the minimum nutrient requirements. If, however, you haven't experienced the benefits you were hoping to experience with your current diet, it may be time to try something new.

Research suggests that, for the vast majority of people, if they were to implement the changes I've described in their diets, they would experience even greater benefit including improved wellness and decreased need for medication.[151]

Putting The Diet To The Test – Case Study

Monica was a 35-year-old female who came to me with concerns of depression for as long as she could remember and compulsive eating. Her depression was only temporarily alleviated by her compulsive eating, after which she would feel physically and emotionally terrible all over again and the cycle would continue.

She had been on different doses of a serotonin–norepinephrine reuptake inhibitor drug for several years, which helped somewhat, but she had self-discontinued by the time she came in to see me. She had also been on psychiatric medication from two other drug classes, but she didn't remember them helping and didn't like the way she had felt on them.

When I met Monica, she described cycles of eating whole foods, feeling extremely depressed, compulsively eating processed foods consisting largely of simple carbohydrates, experiencing temporary relief that was followed by her feeling terrible physically and emotionally, which then led to more compulsive eating until she recovered the motivation necessary to break the cycle and return to a diet of unprocessed foods.

Monica was actively in a cycle of compulsive eating when we met. She reported, however, that when she wasn't eating compulsively, her diet was one that many people would consider to be "clean," consisting of vegetables, fruits, unprocessed meat, seafood, nuts, seeds, and coffee. She was avoiding dairy, grains, soy, other legumes, added sugar, other additives, and highly processed foods.

I ran labs for Monica and, based on her results, her history, and her then-current symptoms, I recommended that she start the P7 Protocol™ Diet along with a few other preliminary recommendations. Monica implemented the dietary changes and started on the other aspects of our preliminary treatment plan. When I followed up with her a little over two weeks later, she reported that she had been feeling significantly better since implementing the plan.

This improvement is likely because Monica's carbohydrate restriction and consumption of a diet comparatively high is protein and fat was negatively impacting serotonin production, whereas when she transitioned to the P7 Protocol™ Diet, her higher carbohydrate intake led to increased transport of tryptophan into the brain which led to increased serotonin production and release in the brain, resulting in reduced carbohydrate cravings and improved mood.[101-102,104]

When we met to discuss Monica's functional medicine test results and further adjust her treatment plan the following month, she reported that she had felt great for several weeks, but noticed that when she deviated from the diet, it quickly led to a downward spiral of depressed mood and compulsive eating. I made recommendations to address the abnormalities that Monica's lab results showed with her neurochemistry, HPA axis, and gastrointestinal flora at that visit in order to further address the cause of her concerns. When I last heard from her, which was about a month after making those adjustments to her treatment plan, she informed me that she had been feeling much better for several weeks and experiencing "massive improvement." She described improved energy, feeling much more emotionally balanced, and being able to keep up with her life again.

CHAPTER TWELVE

How the Trauma Caused the Drama

· · · · · · · · · · · · · · · · · · ·

Traumatic Experiences and Their
Effects on Mental Health

O NGOING RESEARCH CONTINUES TO validate the fact that there is a distinct connection between the emotions we experience in early childhood and our mental health as adults. Some of the most interesting research about this topic, in my opinion, pertains to the connection between childhood trauma, the inflammatory response, and later mental health outcomes. Researchers set out to understand the effect that adverse childhood experiences (ACEs) such as physical, emotional, or sexual abuse, having an incarcerated family member or one who misuses substances, having divorced or separated parents, and other ACEs had on mental health in adulthood.

ACEs and Mental Health Diagnoses

In an effort to uncover the facts, the World Health Organization conducted mental health surveys in over 20 different countries. The results were fascinating. Research demonstrated that people who experienced ACEs were more likely to be diagnosed with mental health concerns including conduct disorder, attention-deficit hyperactivity disorder and oppositional defiant disorder in childhood; and, in adulthood, depression, anxiety disorders (including generalized anxiety disorder, phobias and post-traumatic stress disorder), eating disorders, sexual dysfunction, personality disorder, dissociative disorder, and substance misuse.[152]

Additional research conducted on people from over 16,000 households in South Dakota found that the Native Americans there as a statistical group were more likely to experience ACEs than non-Native Americans. They also found that, for both Native Americans and non-Native Americans, an ACE score of 6 or higher was associated with an increased risk of mental health concerns including depression, anxiety, post-traumatic stress disorder, severe alcohol misuse, and smoking.[153]

Childhood Sexual Abuse and Psychosis

Some of the latest research demonstrates that the link between ACEs, specifically childhood sexual abuse, and psychosis is as strong as or stronger than the link between ACEs and other mental health concerns. In fact, research suggests that if you control for history of hallucinations and delusions in first-degree relatives (e.g. only compare those who do have this family history with each other and those who don't with others who don't), people who were abused as children were on average nine times more likely to experience psychosis than those who weren't. Those who suffered "mild abuse" were twice as likely as the un-abused to experience psychosis later in life, and those who suffered "severe abuse" were over 48 times more likely to experience psychosis later in life. People who were subjected to physical or sexual abuse as children were more likely to be admitted to a psychiatric hospital, have earlier, longer and more frequent admissions, be prescribed more psychiatric medication, self-harm, attempt suicide, and have more severe symptoms.[154]

Scientists and trauma-informed practitioners believe this predisposition to mental illness is partially due to neuro-biological factors such as the inflammatory response. We currently believe that when a person experiences chronic stress as a child, the psychological experiences like abuse and neglect are programmed into the immune system. The macrophages (a type of white blood cell) develop a pro-inflammatory tendency, meaning that they display an exaggerated inflammatory response within the body. This dysregulation of the inflammatory response leads to a chronic "wear and tear" effect on the brain and other organs.[155]

Exposure to chronic stress and the resulting dysregulated immune system induce changes in regions of the developing brain, specifically the amygdala and the hippocampus. These changes affect a variety of different mental functions including regulation of the stress response, attention, memory, planning, and learning new skills.[156]

Scientists also believe that the link between ACEs and mental health disorders is related to neurotransmitter and adrenal function. For example, the traumagenic neurodevelopmental model of psychosis suggests that psychosis may be a direct result of trauma. This claim is founded upon and supported by the fact that researchers observed biochemical and structural similarities between the brains and adrenal glands of traumatized children and adults who were diagnosed with schizophrenia. These similarities include abnormalities of the neurotransmitters dopamine, serotonin, and norepinephrine; structural differences in the brain such as hippocampal damage, cerebral atrophy, ventricular enlargements and reversed cerebral asymmetry; and hyper-reactivity of the HPA axis to stress.[157]

Experiencing physical or emotional neglect; physical, emotional, or sexual abuse; family separation through incarceration, divorce, or death; war; growing up with an addicted or mentally ill family member; or some other unfortunate childhood experience can not only be emotionally traumatizing, but can also have real and serious effects on your physical and mental health. Realizing this fact can be extremely liberating if you're a person who has experienced ACEs. When you realize that the circumstances that you endured in childhood led to your current physical, mental, social, and maybe even spiritual health concerns and helped to make you who you are (both the desirable and the unwanted qualities), it makes it so much easier for you to extend grace to yourself and make sense of your current situation. You no longer need to be impatient with yourself or wonder why you react this way or do certain things; it all makes sense.

While ACEs may have led to a pro-inflammatory tendency in your body and poor physical and mental health, this does not need to continue forever. Once you come to terms with the effects that your ACEs have had on your health and initiate the process of healing through taking specific steps such as what I call "looking back to move forward," you can begin to rewire your brain by making new neuronal connections and creating new thought patterns, resulting in improved overall wellbeing.

As soon as you are ready to do so, you can begin processing your past, looking back in order to move forward. I typically recommend a journaling exercise for my patients where they write down events (or groups of events) that took place in their past and how these events had a formative effect on the person they have become. An example would be, "I was consistently bullied at school because of my disability and this led to me turning inward, fearing to be ridiculed, and being diagnosed with social anxiety disorder and major depression."

I've found that when my patients understand the things that made them who they are, they are better able to predict how they would respond in a given situation and make conscious decisions to redirect their thoughts or respond differently.

Addressing your past is crucial to obtaining healing from traumatic events. In addition to intellectually and emotionally processing the past, I've found finding meaning and purpose in the past to be indispensible on the healing journey. It takes time and energy to get to this place, but I have found that when, for example, a victim of abuse is able to find a sense of purpose in and make sense of his or her experiences by channeling that energy into helping others who are or have been in a similar situation, healing is expedited.

There's always something that you can do. If you can't advocate for others, start a non-profit organization to help, donate to a related cause, or adopt or otherwise support people under similar circumstances, then you can start a blog where you write about your experiences and share words of encouragement to others in similar situations or form a local or virtual support group; the possibilities really are endless.

Another important part of the healing journey is mending and strengthening social ties. It's not always possible to reconcile your relationships with people who have caused you harm; sometimes people become estranged, lose their reasoning capabilities, or even die. If it is possible, however, and this should be decided on a case-by-case basis, it may be of value to try to mend the broken relationship. You should use your discretion in this arena and avoid putting yourself in a situation where you may be harmed or placed in a situation for which you or the person or people you are seeking to reconcile with are not emotionally prepared to handle.

If it isn't possible or in your best interest to try to mend the relationship, I've found writing a letter to the person or people explaining the things that happened between you, how they made you feel, how they affected you and continue to affect you as an adult, and how you are working toward overcoming those experiences to be extremely beneficial. Write to them about your forgiveness for them or your desire to forgive them if you aren't quite there yet. I've found this exercise to be particularly freeing and I trust that you will as well.

In cases where you've tried all of my previous recommendations, and you've started on a protocol to decrease the hyper-reactivity of your HPA axis and address the other physical and mental health concerns associated with your ACEs, but you still feel like you still need more professional help, I highly recommend finding a qualified cognitive behavioral therapist to work with who can help you to process these emotions by recommending cognitive behavioral therapy activities like cognitive restructuring, self-monitoring, and other evidence-based therapies that are calculated to help you move forward and regain your mental wellbeing.

CHAPTER THIRTEEN

Nothing Works Without You

· · · · · · · · · · · · · · · · · ·

*The Importance of Perseverance in
Regaining Mental Wellbeing*

N ow that i've written to you about my P7 Protocol™ for integrated mental wellbeing and shared case studies from a few of my patients, I want to set the record straight. If for any reason while reading this book you got the impression that addressing your mental health using an integrative approach would be easy, I want to correct that thought; in the majority of cases, regaining mental wellness naturally is very hard work, and doing so requires an essential ingredient—perseverance.

If you are currently on medication and your goal is to manage your mental and overall wellbeing using the P7 Protocol™, I want you to know that, while I have had patients come in reporting that they discontinued their psychiatric medication cold-turkey (this is absolutely not recommended, in case that wasn't clear), in most cases weaning off of your medication can be a long and hard road.

For example, SSRI medications like Lexapro and Zoloft can result in what is known clinically as behavioral apathy and emotional blunting.[158] This means that if you're taking an SSRI, you may find that you experience a lack of motivation that isn't explained by your depressed feelings and that you aren't responding as you normally would to emotional stimuli. This could be a reduction in the intensity of emotions or a reduction in your overall range of emotions. These symptoms of indifference tend to come on gradually and intensify on higher doses of medications. I've found that many of my patients don't notice the indifference creeping up on them while taking the medication, but a light bulb goes off when they discontinue the medication and they report being "able to cry again" after discontinuation.

Think about this hypothetical situation—you've wanted to address your concerns using an integrative approach and you've finally begun to experience enough improvement on the P7 Protocol™ to initiate the weaning process. You've wanted to be medication-free and experience improved wellbeing for some time now, and now it seems like your goal is finally within your reach. You've gone through your weaning process and hit a few road bumps, but overall, the process was uneventful. Now you're here. You took the last dosage of your medication 4 days ago, and now, when you expected that you would be feeling amazing, feeling proud of your achievements, and seeing life with new meaning, instead, you can't get out of bed, you're continuously crying whereas you almost never cried before, and you just don't understand what's going on or what you should do.

This is a very real scenario, and I tell you this not to scare or deter you, but to help you to have realistic expectations about the process. The reason this is a very realistic scenario is that while a natural, functional approach provides the body with everything it needs, corrects deficiencies and dysregulated systems, and gently nudges the body in the right direction, pharmaceutical medications, as we've discussed in great detail, impose chemical changes upon your body that can result in a variety of secondary and tertiary effects. Instead of helping the body to do what it needs to do naturally, they force their changes upon the body. This is necessary in some cases, but the unfortunate reality is that when you rely on psychiatric medication to address your concerns and then remove the medication from the equation, at best the body continues to operate in the way it did before you were on the medication, and at worse you return to the same or an even worse mental state and suffer physical effects as well.

Oftentimes when we consent to try pharmaceutical medication, it is because we are experiencing emotional symptoms that we either don't know how to deal with, don't want to deal with, or don't have the time to deal with. When we begin taking the medication, these symptoms, in many cases, appear to resolve. When we discontinue the medication, it's very likely that those emotions that we didn't take the time to process will resurface.

It's similar to this hypothetical situation: someone is coming over and your house isn't clean, so you pick up all of the clothes and other items that are strewn all over your floor and stuff them into a closet. While they are there (e.g. the pharmaceutical is on board), everything appears to be clean and put together, but when they leave, you find that you actually are still left with a messy closet which you need to sort through. It's not that the closet will never be clean and organized; it's just that it takes much more time and effort to organize the closet than it took to stuff everything in there in the first place.

I say that an integrative approach is hard work and requires perseverance because, unless your mental health concern is completely due to a hormonal imbalance like a thyroid problem or some other physical health concern, a large part of regaining healing consists of learning to work through these emotions instead of trying to suppress them.

This process brings about its desired results, but it's not a bed of roses. It takes hard work, effort, time, money, motivation, and determination on your part. For some people, addressing physical health concerns that contribute to their poor mental health leads to a dramatic improvement in their mental and overall wellbeing. For others, giving the body what it needs physically and then discontinuing or reducing their medication brings about the desired results. For others, it takes all of those things, as well as long, hard hours of work, sorting through past experiences and complex emotions, and a variety of different therapies and treatments in order to bring about the desired results.

If you are determined, you make up your mind that now is your time, you're willing to persevere in regaining your mental and overall wellbeing, even when you actually want to quit, and you're ready to put your all into regaining optimal health, then you absolutely can. It may be hard work, but in the end it will be worth it to be able to find true love, reconnect with your spouse, children, or grandchildren, build that business, climb Mount Everest, travel the world, help others who are in the situation you were once in, and have the freedom to live the life that you want to live.

I am confident that if you will put your all into this journey and make the necessary adjustments, cultivate the right mindset, and reach out for help when you need it, you will succeed and the reward on the other side will be so worth it.

References

1. Tavakoli HR. "A closer evaluation of current methods in psychiatric assessments: a challenge for the biopsychosocial model." *Psychiatry (Edgmont)*. 6.2 (2009):25–30.

2. Hirschfeld RM, Lewis L, et al. "Perceptions and Impact of Bipolar Disorder." *Journal of Clinical Psychiatry*. 64.2 (2003), 161–174.

3. Price DM. "For 175 Years: Treating Mentally Ill With Dignity." *The New York Times*, 17 Apr. 1988, www.nytimes.com/1988/04/17/us/for-175-years-treating-mentally-ill-with-dignity.html.

4. Penn Medicine. "Dr. Benjamin Rush." *History of Pennsylvania Hospital*, www.uphs.upenn.edu/paharc/features/brush.html.

5. Whitaker R. *Mad in America*. Perseus Publishing, 2002.

6. Miller AL. "The methylation, neurotransmitter, and antioxidant connections between folate and depression." *Alternative Medicine Review*. 13.3 (2008): 216-226

7. Moustafa AA, Hewedi DH, et al. "Homocysteine levels in schizophrenia and affective disorders—focus on cognition." *Frontiers in Behavioral Neuroscience* 8 (2014): 343. 10.3389/fnbeh.2014.00343

8. Gilbody S, Lewis S, et al. "Methylenetetrahydrofolate reductase (MTHFR) genetic polymorphisms and psychiatric disorders: a HuGE review." *American Journal of Epidemiology*. 165.1 (2007): 1–13 10.1093/aje/kwj347

9. Lynch T, Price A. "The effect of cytochrome P450 metabolism on drug response, interactions and adverse effects." *American Family Physician.* 76.3 (2007):391–396.

10. Anderson S, Panka J, et al. "Anxiety and Methylenetetrahydrofolate Reductase Mutation Treated With S-Adenosyl Methionine and Methylated B Vitamins". *Integrative Medicine (Encinitas, California).* 15.2 (2016):48-52.

11. Valenta LJ, Elias AN, et al. "ACTH Stimulation of Adrenal Epinephrine and Norepinephrine Release." *Hormone research.* 23.1 (1986):16-20. 10.1159/000180283.

12. Jantz G. "Irritable Male Syndrome, It's No Laughing Matter." The Huffington Post, TheHuffingtonPost.com, 24 Mar. 2012, www.huffingtonpost. com/dr-gregory-jantz-phd/irritable-male-syndrome-i_b_1202904.html.

13. Seidman SN. "Normative hypogonadism and depression: Does 'andropause' exist?" *International journal of impotence research.* 18.5 (2006). 415-22. 10.1038/sj.ijir.3901443.

14. Markham JA. "Sex steroids and schizophrenia." *Reviews in Endocrine & Metabolic Disorders.*13.3 (2012):187-207. 10.1007/s11154-011-9184-2.

15. da Silva TL, Ravindran AV. "Contribution of sex hormones to gender differences in schizophrenia: A review." *Asian Journal of Psychiatry.* 18 (2015):2-14. 10.1016/j.ajp.2015.07.016.

16. Studd J. "Severe premenstrual syndrome and bipolar disorder: a tragic confusion." *Menopause International.*18.2 (2012):82–6. 10.1258/ mi.2012.012018.

17. Genovese A, Smith T, et al. "'Is It Her Hormones?': Psychiatric Diagnoses and Polycystic Ovarian Syndrome." *Journal of*

Developmental and Behavioral Pediatrics. 37.1 (2016):103-4. 10.1097/DBP.0000000000000243

18. Munk-Olsen T, Laursen TM, et al. "New parents and mental disorders. A population-based register study." *JAMA*. 296.21 (2006): 2582–9.

19. Spencer CA, Hollowell JG, et al. "National Health and Nutrition Examination Survey III thyroid-stimulating hormone (TSH)-thyroperoxidase antibody relationships demonstrate that TSH upper reference limits may be skewed by occult thyroid dysfunction." *Journal of Clinical Endocrinology and Metabolism*. 92.11 (2007):4236–40. 10.1210/jc.2007-0287

20. Foster JA, McVey Neufeld K-A. "Gut-brain axis: how the microbiome influences anxiety and depression." *Trends in Neurosciences*. 36.5 (2013):305–12. 10.1016/j.tins.2013.01.005

21. Furness JB, Callaghan BP, et al. "The enteric nervous system and gastrointestinal innervation: integrated local and central control." *Advances in Experimental Medicine and Biology*. 817 (2014):39–71. 10.1007/978-1-4939-0897-4_3

22. Gibbens, S. "Are Dogs Smarter Than Cats? Science Has an Answer." National Geographic Society, 30 Nov. 2017, news.nationalgeographic.com/2017/11/dog-cat-brains-neurons-intelligence-study-spd/.

23. Vighi G, Marcucci F, et al. "Allergy and the Gastrointestinal System." *Clinical and Experimental Immunology*. 153 (2008):3–6. 10.1111/j.1365-2249.2008.03713.x

24. Bischoff SC, Barbara G, et al. "Intestinal Permeability – a New Target for Disease Prevention and Therapy." *BMC Gastroenterology* 14 (2014):189

25. Browning KN, Verheijden S, et al. "The vagus nerve in appetite regulation, mood, and intestinal inflammation." *Gastroenterology*. 152.4 (2017):730–744. 10.1053/j.gastro.2016.10.046

26. Breit S, Kupferberg A, et al. "Vagus Nerve as Modulator of the Brain–Gut Axis in Psychiatric and Inflammatory Disorders." *Frontiers in Psychiatry.* 9 (2018): 44. 0.3389/fpsyt.2018.00044

27. Liu X, Cao S, et al. "Modulation of gut microbiota-brain axis by probiotics, prebiotics, and diet." *Journal of Agricultural and Food Chemistry.* 63.36 (2015):7885–95. 10.1021/acs.jafc.5b02404

28. Bravo JA, Forsythe P, et al. "Ingestion of Lactobacillus strain regulates emotional behavior and central GABA receptor expression in a mouse via the vagus nerve." *Proceedings of the National Academy of Sciences of the USA.* 108.38 (2011), 16050–5. 10.1073/pnas.1102999108

29. Wang B, Yao M, et al. "The Human Microbiota in Health and Disease." *Engineering.* 3.1 (2017):71-82. 10.1016/J.ENG.2017.01.008

30. Abraham BP, Kane S. "Fecal markers: calprotectin and lactoferrin." *Gastroenterology Clinics of North America.* 41.2 (2012):483–95. 10.1016/j.gtc.2012.01.007

31. Yamamoto T, Shiraki M, et al. "Faecal Calprotectin and Lactoferrin as Markers for Monitoring Disease Activity and Predicting Clinical Recurrence in Patients with Crohn's Disease after Ileocolonic Resection: A Prospective Pilot Study." *United European Gastroenterology Journal* 1.5 (2013): 368-74. 10.1177/2050640613501818.

32. Schnorr SL, Bachner HA. "Integrative Therapies in Anxiety Treatment with Special Emphasis on the Gut Microbiome." *The Yale Journal of Biology and Medicine.* 89.3 (2016): 397–422.

33. Jaglin M, Rhimi M, et al. "Indole, a Signaling Molecule Produced by the Gut Microbiota, Negatively Impacts Emotional Behaviors in Rats." *Frontiers in Neuroscience.* 216 :(2018) 12. 10.3389/fnins.2018.00216

34. Guertzel MN. "Escherichia, Klebsiella, Enterobacter, Serratia, Citrobacter, and Proteus." In: Baron S, editor. Medical Microbiology. 4th edition. Galveston (TX): University of Texas Medical Branch at Galveston; 1996. Chapter 26. Available from: https://www.ncbi.nlm.nih.gov/books/NBK8035/

35. Lyte M., Li W, et al. "Induction of anxiety-like behavior in mice during the initial stages of infection with the agent of murine colonic hyperplasia *Citrobacter rodentium*." *Physiology & Behavior.*89.3 (2006): 350–7. 10.1016/j.physbeh.2006.06.019.

36. Bland J. "Intestinal Microbiome, Akkermansia Muciniphila, and Medical Nutrition Therapy." *Integrative Medicine: A Clinician's Journal* 15.5 (2016): 14–16.

37. Zaporozhets TS, Besednova NN, et al. "The prebiotic potential of polysaccharides and extracts of seaweeds." *Russian Journal of Marine Biology.* 40.1 (2014): 1-9. 10.1134/S1063074014010106

38. Beyer KM, Kaltenbach A, et al. "Exposure to Neighborhood Green Space and Mental Health: Evidence from the Survey of the Health of Wisconsin." *International Journal of Environmental Research and Public Health.* 11.3 (2014): 3453–72. 10.3390/ijerph110303453

39. Maas J, Verheij RA, et al. "Morbidity is related to a green living environment." *Journal of Epidemiology & Community Health* 63.12 (2009):967-73. 10.1136/jech.2008.079038

40. Ellett L, Freeman D, et al. "The psychological effect of an urban environment on individuals with persecutory delusions: The Camberwell walk study." *Schizophrenia Research.* 99.1-3 (2008): 77–84. 10.1016/j.schres.2007.10.027

41. Freeman D, Emsley R, et al. "The Stress of the Street for Patients With Persecutory Delusions: A Test of the Symptomatic and Psychological

Effects of Going Outside Into a Busy Urban Area." *Schizophrenia bulletin.* 41.4 (2014): 971-9. 10.1093/schbul/sbu173.

42. Carek PJ, Laibstain SE, et al. "Exercise for the treatment of depression and anxiety." *International Journal of Psychiatry in Medicine.* 41.1 (2011), 15–28. 10.2190/PM.41.1.c

43. Sleiman SF, Henry J, et al. "Exercise Promotes the Expression of Brain Derived Neurotrophic Factor (BDNF) through the Action of the Ketone Body B-Hydroxybutyrate." *eLife.* 5 (2016): e15092. 10.7554/eLife.15092

44. Mittal VA, Vargas T, et al. "Exercise treatments for psychosis: a review." *Current Treatment Options in Psychiatry.* 4.2 (2017):152–66. 10.1007/s40501-017-0112-2

45. Mackay G, Neill J. "The effect of 'green exercise' on state anxiety and the role of exercise duration, and greenness: a quasi-experimental study." *Psychology of Sport and Exercise.* 11.3 (2010), 238–45. 10.1016/j.psychsport.2010.01.002

46. Sims-Gould J, Vazirian S, et al. "Jump step - a community based participatory approach to physical activity & mental wellness." *BMC Psychiatry.* 17.1 (2017): 319. 10.1186/s12888-017-1476-y.

47. Caddick N, Smith B. "The impact of sport and physical activity on the well-being of combat veterans: a systematic review." *Psychology of Sport and Exercise.* 15.1 (2014): 9-18. 10.1016/j.psychsport.2013.09.011

48. Roe J. "Cities, Green Space, and Mental Well-Being." *Oxford Research Encyclopedia of Environmental Science.* 2016-11-22. Oxford University Press. 10.1093/acrefore/9780199389414.013.93

49. Krysta K, Krzystanek M, et al. "Sleep and Inflammatory Markers in Different Psychiatric Disorders." *Journal of Neural Transmission (Vienna)*. 124.Suppl 1 (2017): 179–86. 10.1007/s00702-015-1492-3

50. Allison KC, Spaeth A, et al. "Sleep and eating disorders." *Current Psychiatry Report*. 18.10 (2016): 92. 10.1007/s11920-016-0728-8.

51. Poznanski B, Cornacchio D, et al. "The Link Between Anxiety Severity and Irritability Among Anxious Youth: Evaluating the Mediating Role of Sleep Problems." *Child Psychiatry & Human Development*. 49.2 (2017): 352-9. 10.1007/s10578-017-0769-1.

52. McMakin DL, Alfano CA. "Sleep and Anxiety in Late Childhood and Early Adolescence." *Current opinion in psychiatry*. 28.6 (2015): 483–9. 10.1097/YCO.0000000000000204

53. Harandi TF, Taghinasab MM, et al. "The Correlation of Social Support with Mental Health: A Meta-Analysis." *Electronic Physician*. 9.9 (2017): 5212–22. 10.19082/5212.

54. Riahi MA, Verdinia AA, et al. "Relationship between social support and mental health." *Social Welfare Quarterly*. 10.39 (2011):85–121.

55. Santos PR, Capote Júnior JRFG, et al. "Religious Coping Methods Predict Depression and Quality of Life among End-Stage Renal Disease Patients Undergoing Hemodialysis: a Cross-Sectional Study." *BMC Nephrology*. 18.1 (2017):197. 10.1186/s12882-017-0619-1.

56. Sharma V, Marin DB, et al. "Religion, Spirituality, and Mental Health of U.S. Military Veterans: Results from the National Health and Resilience in Veterans Study." *Journal of Affective Disorders*. 217 (2017): 197–204. 10.1016/j.jad.2017.03.071.

57. Smith-MacDonald L, Norris JM, et al. "Spirituality and Mental Well-Being in Combat Veterans: A Systematic Review." *Military Medicine*. 182.11 (2017): e1920-e1940. 10.7205/milmed-d-17-00099.

58. Tsitsas GD, Paschali AA. "A Cognitive-Behavior Therapy Applied to a Social Anxiety Disorder and a Specific Phobia, Case Study." *Health Psychology Research*. 2.3 (2014):1603. 10.4081/hpr.2014.1603.

59. "DailyMed - SEROQUEL- Quetiapine Fumarate Tablet, Film Coated." *U.S. National Library of Medicine*, National Institutes of Health, 23 Feb. 2017, dailymed.nlm.nih.gov/dailymed/drugInfo.cfm?setid=0584dda8-bc3c-48fe-1a90-79608f78e8a0.

60. "DailyMed - ZOLOFT- Sertraline Hydrochloride Tablet, Film Coated ZOLOFT- Sertraline Hydrochloride Solution, Concentrate." U.S. National Library of Medicine, National Institutes of Health, 23 Apr. 2018, dailymed.nlm.nih.gov/dailymed/drugInfo.cfm?setid=-fe9e8b7d-61ea-409d-84aa-3ebd79a046b5.

61. Abe C, Ekman CJ, et al. "Manic episodes are related to changes in frontal cortex: a longitudinal neuroimaging study of bipolar disorder 1." *Brain* 138.11 (2015): 3440–48. 10.1093/brain/awv266

62. Breggin PR. "Psychiatric drug-induced Chronic Brain Impairment (CBI): implications for long-term treatment with psychiatric medication." *International Journal of Risk and Safety in Medicine*. 23.4 (2011):193–200. 10.3233/JRS-2011-0542

63. Flock J. "Oprah Accused of Whipping up Anti-Beef 'Lynch Mob'." *CNN*, Cable News Network, 21 Jan. 1998. cnn.com/US/9801/21/oprah.beef/.

64. Usborne D. "Oprah Triumphs over the Texas Cattle Ranchers." *The Independent*, Independent Digital News and Media, 27 Feb. 1998, independent.co.uk/news/oprah-triumphs-over-the-texas-cattle-ranchers-1147137.html.

65. Duke University. "Introduction to Evidence-Based Practice: Types of Studies." *Duke University Medical Center Library & Archives*, 8 Mar. 2018, guides.mclibrary.duke.edu/ebmtutorial/study-types.

66. Lai JS, Hiles S,et al. "A systematic review and meta-analysis of dietary patterns and depression in community-dwelling adults." *The American Journal of Clinical Nutrition*. 99.1 (2014): 181–197. 10.3945/ajcn.113.069880

67. Cartwright N. "What are randomised controlled trials good for?" *Philosophical Studies*. 147 (2010): 59. 10.1007/s11098-009-9450-2

68. Li Y, Lv M-R, et al. "Dietary patterns and depression risk: a meta-analysis." *Psychiatry Research*. 253 (2017): 373–82. 10.1016/j.psychres.2017.04.020

69. Beezhold BL, Johnston CS. "Restriction of meat, fish, and poultry in omnivores improves mood: a pilot randomized controlled trial." *Nutrition Journal*. 11 (2012): 9–15. 10.1186/1475-2891-11-9.

70. Carlsen MH, Halvorsen BL, et al. "The total antioxidant content of more than 3100 foods, beverages, spices, herbs and supplements used worldwide." *Nutrition Journal*. 9.3 (2010): 3. 10.1186/1475-2891-9-3.

71. Salim S. "Oxidative Stress and Psychological Disorders." *Current Neuropharmacology* 12.2 (2014): 140–147. 10.2174/1570159X11666131120230309

72. Pandya CD, Howell KR, et al. "Antioxidants as potential therapeutics for neuropsychiatric disorders." *Prog Neuropsychopharmacol Biol Psychiatry*. 46 (2013):214–223. 10.1016/j.pnpbp.2012.10.017

73. Gautam M, Agrawal M, et al. "Role of antioxidants in generalised anxiety disorder and depression." *Indian Journal of Psychiatry*. 54 (2012): 244-7. 10.4103/0019-5545.102424

74. Kocot J, Luchowska-Kocot D, et al. "Does Vitamin C Influence Neurodegenerative Diseases and Psychiatric Disorders?" *Nutrients.* 9.7 (2017): 659. 10.3390/nu9070659

75. Szeto YT, Kwok TC, et al. "Effects of a long-term vegetarian diet on biomarkers of antioxidant status and cardiovascular disease risk." *Nutrition.* 20.10 (2004):863–6. 10.1016/j.nut.2004.06.006.

76. Saneei P, Esmaillzadeh A, et al. "Combined healthy lifestyle is inversely associated with psychological disorders among adults." *PLoS ONE.* 11 (2016):e0146888. 10.1371/journal.pone.0146888.

77. Payne ME, Steck SE, et al. "Fruit, vegetable, and antioxidant intakes are lower in older adults with depression." *Journal of the Academy of Nutrition and Dietetics.* 112.12 (2012): 2022–7. 10.1016/j.jand.2012.08.026.

78. Litalien C, Beaulieu P. "Chapter 117 - Molecular Mechanisms of Drug Actions: From Receptors to Effectors," In *Pediatric Critical Care* (Fourth Edition), edited by Bradley P. Fuhrman and Jerry J. Zimmerman, Mosby, Saint Louis, 2011, Pages 1553-1568, ISBN 9780323073073, 10.1016/B978-0-323-07307-3.10117-X.

79. Kim YJ, Chung HY. "Antioxidative and anti-inflammatory actions of docosahexaenoic acid and eicosapentaenoic acid in renal epithelial cells and macrophages." *Journal of Medicinal Food.* 10.2 (2007):225–31. 10.1089/jmf.2006.092.

80. Farooqui AA, Horrocks LA, et al. "Modulation of inflammation in brain: a matter of fat." *Journal of Neurochemistry.* 101.3 (2007): 577–99. 10.1111/j.1471-4159.2006.04371.x

81. Kidd PM. "Omega-3 DHA and EPA for cognition, behavior, and mood: clinical findings and structural-functional synergies with cell membrane phospholipids." *Alternative Medicine Review.* 12.3 (2007): 207–27.

82. Hashimoto K, Shimizu E, et al. "Critical role of brain-derived neuro-trophic factor in mood disorders." *Brain Research Brain Research Reviews.* 45.2 (2004):104–14. 10.1016/j.brainresrev.2004.02.003

83. Stahl L, Begg D, et al. "The role of omega-3 fatty acids in mood disorders." *Current Opinion in Investigational Drugs.* 9.1 (2008): 57–64.

84. Aranda N, Valls RM, et al. (2017). "Consumption of seafood and its estimated heavy metals are associated with lipid profile and oxidative lipid damage on healthy adults from a Spanish Mediterranean area: A cross-sectional study." *Environmental research.* 155 (2017). 644-51. 10.1016/j.envres.2017.04.037.

85. Brinkel J, Khan MH, et al. "A systematic review of arsenic exposure and its social and mental health effects with special reference to Bangladesh. " *International Journal of Environmental Research and Public Health.* 6.5 (2009):1609–19. 10.3390/ijerph6051609.

86. Kern JK, Geier DA, et al. "Evidence supporting a link between dental amalgams and chronic illness, fatigue, depression, anxiety, and suicide." *Neuro Endocrinology Letters.* 35.7 (2014): 537–52.

87. Troiano G, Mercurio I, et al. "Suicide behaviour and arsenic levels in drinking water: a possible association?" *Egyptian journal of forensic sciences.* 7.1 (2017): 2. 10.1186/s41935-017-0005-y

88. Sarter B, Kelsey KS, et al. "Blood docosahexaenoic acid and eicosap-entaenoic acid in vegans: associations with age and gender and effects of an algal-derived omega-3 fatty acid supplement." *Clinical Nutrition.* 34.2 (2015):212–8. 10.1016/j.clnu.2014.03.003

89. Simopoulos AP. "The importance of the ratio of omega-6/omega-3 essential fatty acids." *Biomedicine & Pharmacotherapy.* 56.8 (2002): 365–79. 10.1016/S0753-3322(02)00253-6.

90. Adam O, Tesche A, et al. "Impact of linoleic acid intake on arachidonic acid formation and eicosanoid biosynthesis in humans." *Prostaglandins Leukotrienes and Essential Fatty Acids.* 79 (2008): 177-81. 10.1016/j.plefa.2008.09.007

91. Saunders AV, Davis BC, et al. "Omega-3 polyunsaturated fatty acids and vegetarian diets." *Medical Journal of Australia.* 199.4 (2013): 22-6. 10.5694/mja11.11507

92. Rodriguez-Leyva D, Dupasquier CMC, et al. "The cardiovascular effects of flaxseed and its omega-3 fatty acid, alpha-linolenic acid." *Canadian Journal of Cardiology.* 26.9 (2010): 489-96.

93. Zeilmaker MJ, Hoekstra J, et al. "Fish consumption during child bearing age: A quantitative risk–benefit analysis on neurodevelopment." *Food and Chemical Toxicology.* 54 (2013): 30–4. 10.1016/j.fct.2011.10.068.

94. Glynn A, Aune M, et al. "Determinants of serum concentrations of organochlorine compounds in Swedish pregnant women: A cross-sectional study." *Environmental Health.* 6 (2007):2. 10.1186/1476-069X-6-2.

95. Katcher HI, Ferdowsian HR, et al. "A worksite vegan nutrition program is well-accepted and improves health-related quality of life and work productivity." *Annals of Nutrition and Metabolism.* 56.4 (2010):245–52. 10.1159/000288281.

96. Agarwal U, Mishra S, et al. "A multicenter randomized controlled trial of a nutrition intervention program in a multiethnic adult population in the corporate setting reduces depression and anxiety and improves quality of life: the GEICO study." *American Journal of Health Promotion.* 29.4 (2015): 245-54. 10.4278/ajhp.130218-QUAN-72

97. Buettner D. "Loma Linda, California: A Group of Americans Living 10 Years Longer." *Blue Zones*®. bluezones.com/exploration/loma-linda-california/.

98. Beezhold BL, Johnston CS, et al. "Vegetarian diets are associated with healthy mood states: a cross-sectional study in Seventh-day Adventist adults." *Nutrition Journal.* 9 (2010):26. 10.1186/1475-2891-9-26.

99. Lucas M, Mirzaei F, et al. "Dietary intake of n-3 and n-6 fatty acids and the risk of clinical depression in women: a 10-y prospective follow-up study." *American Journal of Clinical Nutrition.* 93 (2011):1337–43. 10.3945/ajcn.111.011817

100. Brinkworth GD, Buckley JD, et al. "Long-term effects of a very low-carbohydrate diet and a low-fat diet on mood and cognitive function." *Archives of Internal Medicine.* 169.20 (2009):1873–80. 10.1001/archinternmed.2009.329.

101. Wurtman J, Brzezinski A, et al. "Effect of nutrient intake on premenstrual depression." *American Journal of Obstetrics and Gynecology.* 161.5 (1989):1228–34. 10.1016/0002-9378(89)90671-6.

102. Wurtman RJ, Wurtman JJ, et al. "Effects of normal meals rich in carbohydrates or proteins on plasma tryptophan and tyrosine ratios." *The American Journal of Clinical Nutrition.* 77.1 (2003): 128–32. 10.1093/ajcn/77.1.128

103. Yoon M-S. "The Emerging Role of Branched-Chain Amino Acids in Insulin Resistance and Metabolism." *Nutrients.* 8.7 (2016): 405. 10.3390/nu8070405.

104. Hudson, Craig W. et al. "Protein-source tryptophan as an efficacious treatment for social anxiety disorder: a pilot study" *Canadian journal of physiology and pharmacology.* 85.9 (2007): 928–32. 10.1139/Y07-082

105. Levine ME, Suarez JA, et al. "Low protein intake is associated with a major reduction in IGF-1, cancer, and overall mortality in the 65 and younger but not older population." *Cell Metabolism.* 19.3 (2014): 407–17. 10.1016/j.cmet.2014.02.006.

106. Rizzo NS, Jaceldo-Siegl K, et al. "Nutrient profiles of vegetarian and non-vegetarian dietary patterns." *Journal of the Academy of Nutrition and Dietetics.* 113.12 (2013): 1610–9. 10.1016/j.jand.2013.06.349.

107. Nachbar MS, Oppenheim JD. "Lectins in the United States diet: a survey of lectins in commonly consumed foods and a review of the literature." *American Journal of Clinical Nutrition.* 33.11 (1980):2338–45. 10.1093/ajcn/33.11.2338.

108. Freed DL. "Do dietary lectins cause disease?" *BMJ: British Medical Journal.* 318.7190 (1999):1023-1024.

109. Noah ND, Bender AE, et al. "Food poisoning from raw red kidney beans." *British Medical Journal.* 281.6234 (1980): 236–7.

110. Rodhouse JC, Haugh CA, et al. "Red kidney bean poisoning in the UK: an analysis of 50 suspected incidents between 1976 and 1989." *Epidemiology and Infection.* 105.3 (1990):485–491.

111. Pusztai A, Grant G. "Assessment of lectin inactivation by heat and digestion." *Methods in Molecular Medicine.* 9 (1998): 505–14. 10.1385/0-89603-396-1:505.

112. Pal RS, Bhartiya A, et al. "Effect of dehulling, germination and cooking on nutrients, anti-nutrients, fatty acid composition and antioxidant properties in lentil (Lens culinaris)." *Journal of Food Science and Technology.* 54.4 (2017): 909-20. 10.1007/s13197-016-2351-4

113. Lajolo F, Genovese M. "Nutritional Significance of Lectins and Enzyme Inhibitors from Legumes." *Journal of Agricultural and Food Chemistry.* 50.22 (2002): 6592-8. 10.1021/jf020191k.

114. Graf E, Eaton JW. "Antioxidant functions of phytic acid." *Free Radical Biology and Medicine.* 8.1 (1990): 61–9.

115. Navert B, Sandstrom B, et al. "Reduction of the Phytate Content of Bran by Leavening in Bread and Its Effect on Zinc-Absorption in Man." *British Journal of Nutrition.* 53.1 (1985):47–53. 10.1079/BJN19850009.

116. Tatsinkou Fossi, Bertrand & Akwanwi, Che & Nchanji, Gordon Takop & Ebenye, Yvone & , Bille & Wanji, Samuel. (2016). Phytic acid degradation by selected lactobacilli isolated from fruits and vegetables and their potential as probiotics. *European Journal of Biotechnology and Bioscience.* 4.7 (2016): 34-41.

117. Valachovicova M, Krajcovicova-Kudlackova M, et al. "No evidence of insulin resistance in normal weight vegetarians. A case control study." *European Journal of Nutrition.* 45.1 (2006):52–4. 10.1007/s00394-005-0563-x

118. Kuo CS, Lai NS, et al. "Insulin sensitivity in Chinese ovo-lactovegetarians compared with omnivores." *European Journal of Clinical Nutrition.* 58.2 (2004):312–6. 10.1038/sj.ejcn.1601783.

119. Hung CJ, Huang PC, et al. "Taiwanese vegetarians have higher insulin sensitivity than omnivores." *British Journal of Nutrition.* 95.1 (2006): 129–35. 10.1079/BJN20051588.

120. De Koning L, Fung TT, et al. "Low-carbohydrate diet scores and risk of type 2 diabetes in men." *American Journal of Clinical Nutrition.* 93.4 (2011): 844–50. 10.3945/ajcn.110.004333.

121. Gibson RS, Heath A-L, et al. "Is iron and zinc nutrition a concern for vegetarian infants and young children in industrialized countries?" *The American Journal of Clinical Nutrition.* 100.1(2014): 459–68. 10.3945/ajcn.113.071241

122. Hunt JR. "Moving Toward a Plant-based Diet: Are Iron and Zinc at Risk?" *Nutrition Reviews.* 60.5 (2002):127–34. 10.1301/00296640260093788.

123. Burckhardt P. "The role of low acid load in vegetarian diet on bone health: A narrative review." *Swiss Medical Weekly.* 146 (2016): w14277. 10.4414/smw.2016.14277.

124. Hoogendijk WJG, Lips P, et al. "Depression Is Associated With Decreased 25-Hydroxyvitamin D and Increased Parathyroid Hormone Levels in Older Adults." *Archives of General Psychiatry.* 65.5 (2008):508–12. 10.1001/archpsyc.65.5.508

125. McGrath J, Saari K, et al. "Vitamin D supplementation during the first year of life and risk of schizophrenia: a Finnish birth cohort study." *Schizophrenia Research.* 67.2–3 (2004): 237–45. 10.1016/j.schres.2003.08.005

126. Krause M, Klit A, et al. "Sunscreens: Are They Beneficial for Health? An Overview of Endocrine Disrupting Properties of UV-Filters." *International Journal of Andrology.* 35.3 (2012): 424–36. 10.1111/j.1365-2605.2012.01280.x

127. Ruszkiewicz, JA, Pinkas A, et al. "Neurotoxic Effect of Active Ingredients in Sunscreen Products, a Contemporary Review." *Toxicology Reports.* 4 (2017): 245–59. 10.1016/j.toxrep.2017.05.006.

128. Holick MF, Binkley NC. "Evaluation, Treatment, and Prevention of Vitamin D Deficiency: an Endocrine Society Clinical Practice Guideline." *Journal of Clinical Endocrinology & Metabolism.* 96.7 (2011): 1911–30. 10.1210/jc.2011-0385

129. Ginde AA, Liu MC, et al. "Demographic Differences and Trends of Vitamin D Insufficiency in the US Population, 1988-2004." *Archives of Internal Medicine.* 169.6 (2009):626–32. 10.1001/archinternmed.2008.604

130. Johnson LE. "Vitamin B 12 - Disorders of Nutrition - Merck Manuals Consumer Version." *Merck Manuals Professional Edition*, Merck Manual, merckmanuals.com/home/disorders-of-nutrition/vitamins/vitamin-b-12.

131. Rizzo G, Laganà AS, et al. "Vitamin B12 among Vegetarians: Status, Assessment and Supplementation." *Nutrients*. 8.12 (2016):767. 10.3390/nu8120767.

132. Melina V, Craig W, et al. "Position of the academy of nutrition and dietetics: Vegetarian diets." *Journal of the Academy of Nutrition and Dietetics*. 116.12 (2016): 1970–80. 10.1016/j.jand.2016.09.025

133. Tiwari A, Aggarwal A, et al. "Cooking at Home: A Strategy to Comply With U.S. Dietary Guidelines at No Extra Cost." *American Journal of Preventive Medicine*. 52.5 (2017): 616–24. 10.1016/j.amepre.2017.01.017

134. Brookie KL, Best GI, et al. "Intake of Raw Fruits and Vegetables Is Associated With Better Mental Health Than Intake of Processed Fruits and Vegetables." *Frontiers in Psychology*. 9 (2018): 487. 10.3389/fpsyg.2018.00487

135. Dawson SL, Dash SR, et al. "The importance of diet and gut health to the treatment and prevention of mental disorders." *International Review of Neurobiology*. 131 (2016): 325–46. 10.1016/bs.irn.2016.08.009

136. David LA, Maurice CF, et al. "Diet rapidly and reproducibly alters the human gut microbiome." *Nature*. 505 (2014): 559–63. 10.1038/nature12820

137. Purohit V, Bode JC, et al. "Alcohol, intestinal bacterial growth, intestinal permeability to endotoxin, and medical consequences: summary of a symposium." *Alcohol*. 42.5 (2008):349–61. 10.1016/j.alcohol.2008.03.131.

138. Engen PA, Green SJ, et al. "The gastrointestinal microbiome: alcohol effects on the composition of intestinal microbiota." *Alcohol Research: current reviews*. 37.2 (2015): 223–36.

139. Gage SH, Munafò MR. "Smoking as a causal risk factor for schizophrenia." *Lancet Psychiatry*. 2.9 (2015):778–9. 10.1016/S2215-0366(15)00333-8.

140. Gurillo P, Jauhar S, et al. "Does tobacco use cause psychosis? Systematic review and meta-analysis." *Lancet Psychiatry.* 2 (2015): 718-25. 10.1016/S2215-0366(15)00152-2.

141. Ostacher MJ, LeBeau RT, et al. "Cigarette smoking is associated with suicidality in bipolar disorder." *Bipolar Disorders.* 11.7 (2009):766–71. 10.1111/j.1399-5618.2009.00744.x

142. Lee K-J. "Current smoking and secondhand smoke exposure and depression among Korean adolescents: analysis of a national cross-sectional survey." *BMJ Open.* 4 (2014): e003734. 10.1136/bmjopen-2013-003734.

143. Lara DR. "Caffeine, mental health, and psychiatric disorders." *Journal of Alzheimers Disease.* 20 (2010): 239–48. 10.3233/JAD-2010-1378.

144. Broderick P, Benjamin AB. "Caffeine and psychiatric symptoms: a review." *Journal of the Oklahoma State Medical Association.* 97.12 (2004): 538-42.

145. Lucas M, Mirzaei F, et al. "Coffee, Caffeine, and Risk of Depression Among Women." *Archives of Internal Medicine.* 171.17 (2011): 1571–8. 10.1001/archinternmed.2011.393.

146. Kawachi I, Willett WC, et al. "A Prospective Study of Coffee Drinking and Suicide in Women." *Archives of Internal Medicine.* 156.5 (1996):521–5. 10.1001/archinte.1996.00440050067008.

147. Broderick PJ, Benjamin A, et al. "Caffeine and psychiatric medication interactions: a review." *The Journal of the Oklahoma State Medical Association.* 98.8 (2005). 380-4.

148. Taylor G, Taylor A, et al. "Does smoking reduction worsen mental health? A comparison of two observational approaches." *BMJ Open,* 5.5 (2015): e007812. 10.1136/bmjopen-2015-007812

149. Mendelsohn CP, Kirby DP, et al. "Smoking and mental illness. An update for psychiatrists." *Australasian Psychiatry.* 23.1 (2015):37–43. 10.1177/1039856214562076.

150. Krebs-Smith SM, Guenther PM, et al. "Americans do not meet federal dietary recommendations." *The Journal of Nutrition.* 140.10 (2010): 1832–8. 10.3945/jn.110.124826

151. Tuso PJ, Ismail MH, et al. "Nutritional update for physicians: Plant-based diets." *Permanente Journal.* 17.2 (2013): 61–6. 10.7812/TPP/12-085.

152. Kessler RC, McLaughlin KA, et al. "Childhood adversities and adult psychopathology in the WHO World Mental Health Surveys." *British Journal of Psychiatry.* 197.5 (2010): 378–85. 10.1192/bjp.bp.110.080499.

153. Warne D, Dulacki K, et al. "Adverse Childhood Experiences (ACE) among American Indians in South Dakota and Associations with Mental Health Conditions, Alcohol Use, and Smoking." *Journal of Health Care for the Poor and Underserved.* 28.4 (2017): 1559-77. 10.1353/hpu.2017.0133.

154. Read J, Bentall RP. "Negative Childhood Experiences and Mental Health: Theoretical, Clinical and Primary Prevention Implications." *British Journal of Psychiatry*, 200.2 (2012): 89–91. 10.1192/bjp.bp.111.096727.

155. Miller GE, Chen E, et al. "Psychological stress in childhood and susceptibility to the chronic diseases of aging: Moving toward a model of behavioral and biological mechanisms." *Psychological Bulletin.* 137.6 (2011): 959–97. 10.1037/a0024768.

156. Metzler M, Merrick MT, et al. "Adverse childhood experiences and life opportunities: Shifting the narrative." *Children and Youth Services Review.* 72 (2017): 141-9. 10.1016/j.childyouth.2016.10 021.

157. Read J, Bentall RP. "Negative childhood experiences and mental health: theoretical, clinical and primary prevention implications." *British Journal of Psychiatry*. 200.2 (2012): 89–91. 10.1192/bjp.bp.111.096727

158. Sansone RA, Sansone LA. "SSRI-Induced Indifference." *Psychiatry (Edgmont)* 7.10 (2010): 14–18.

About the Author

D R. JANELLE LOUIS IS a licensed, naturopathic physician and the developer of the P7 Protocol™ for integrated mental wellness. Dr. Louis pursued her ND degree at Southwest College of Naturopathic Medicine and Health Sciences in the state of Arizona. She currently practices at Focus Integrative Healthcare, a functional medicine practice in Atlanta, Georgia.

Dr. Louis has helped patients battling mental health conditions and substance abuse at several recovery clinics to regain their mental and physical health. She has also worked with one of Arizona's top developmental pediatricians helping to assess and treat children with ADHD, autism, and other developmental disorders. Her patients appreciate her ability to apply her knowledge of both pharmaceutical medication and natural therapeutics to their unique situations to help them reach their health goals.

Dr. Louis enjoys providing exceptional, patient-focused care to individuals from all walks of life. She loves helping people to optimize their health naturally and to live radiantly! When she is not practicing medicine, Dr. Louis enjoys spending time with her husband and son, writing, teaching, traveling, and camping.